Discover the Hay Diet Secrets: Unlock total body and mind happiness for better health, weight loss and digestive disorders

Written by the author who has who has 35 years' experience of the Hay Diet

BY:

ROBERT JOHNSTONE

COPYRIGHT © 2025

Notice of Copyright

Written by:

Robert Johnstone

Printing Year, 2025

Table of Contents

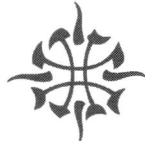

Dr. William Howard Hay

This diet is not something I invented. It began with the work of Dr. William Howard Hay, an American physician who, after suffering a severe breakdown in his own health, changed the course of his life and medicine. He was diagnosed with high blood pressure, kidney disease, and a dilated heart, conditions that modern medicine couldn't seem to fix. At his worst, he weighed 225 pounds and couldn't sleep lying down due to fluid retention. Doctors offered him little hope. So, he took matters into his own hands.

Dr. Hay carefully examined his lifestyle, particularly his eating habits, and reached a radical conclusion for his time: the problem was not what he was eating, but how he was combining his foods. He eliminated poor food combinations, stopped eating incompatible meals like meat with bread or sugar-laden snacks with coffee, and began eating simple, properly combined meals. Within weeks, the changes were undeniable. His weight dropped, his symptoms vanished, and his energy returned.

He went on to spend the next two decades refining and teaching what became known as the Hay Diet, or the Food Combining system. His theory was that the body digests protein and carbohydrate foods in different environments (one acidic, the other alkaline) and that combining both in the same meal forces the body into internal conflict.

Dr. Hay gave up surgery and devoted his life to studying diet, healing patients naturally, and showing that proper eating could be more powerful than medicine. What you'll read in this book is a modern, practical continuation of his philosophy; simplified, updated for today's world, but grounded in the same core truth he discovered:

"Man is an exact composite of what he eats daily, yearly, and as a life habit."

— Dr William Howard Hay

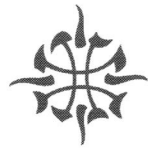

About The Author

Robert Johnstone was born on a Scottish hill farm in the late 1950s and later moved with his family to a farm near Stowmarket in Suffolk, England, where he farmed the land alongside his father. After farming for several years, he opened a lucrative paintball games site in 1989, which he ran successfully until 1997.

Around 1990, while still running the paintball site, he first came across the **Hay Diet**, and it completely changed his life.

Later, he went on to work for Sheikh Hamdan Al Maktoum of the Dubai royal family, managing the Sheikh's 6,000-acre estate near Thetford in South Norfolk. He worked there for over 20 years, and throughout that entire time, he didn't take a single sick day.

Robert has now been following the Hay Diet for 35 years and has never had a bad day on it. He firmly believes that **Hay Diet** is the reason he has stayed fit, healthy, and mentally sharp for so long. He has kept a stable weight of 161 lbs and keeps active by going on brisk walks through the forest near his home. He's genuinely content, always smiling, and full of life.

This is his first book, written to share what has worked for him, and possibly help others looking for a simpler, healthier way to eat and live. Readers are welcome to reach out with questions via the email provided at the end of the book.

Introduction: The Illusion of Self

Let's get one thing straight from the beginning, your body is built on what you feed it. It doesn't matter how many hours you spend at the gym, how many fancy supplements you take, or how "clean" you think your food looks. If you're still combining the wrong foods at every meal, your digestion will suffer. And when your digestion suffers, everything else goes downhill with it, your weight, your mood, your energy, even your skin.

You've probably heard people talk about the 80/20 rule. They usually say it like this: 80 percent of how your body looks and feels is down to what you eat, and only 20 percent comes from exercise. And honestly, after 35 years of living this diet, I'd argue that number might even be higher. Because when your meals are working with your body instead of against it, you don't just slim down, you wake up feeling light, clear, and pain-free.

What most people don't realise is that every single cell in your body gets replaced over time. Roughly every seven to nine years, you're walking around in an entirely new version of yourself, on a cellular level. That means the choices you make today are literally building the future version of you. So if your current cells are inflamed, overloaded, or sluggish from years of poor digestion, imagine what could happen if you gave your body the food it actually knew how to process. Not just occasionally, but consistently.

That's why this isn't just a diet. It's a decision to take responsibility for what goes on your plate. You don't need to change who you are; you just need to change how your meals are built.

And that's where the Hay Diet comes in.

It isn't some polished breakdown of food science with pages of footnotes either. It's a straight-up guide to what I've learned from actually doing this diet for decades. I've gone out to meals, travelled, cooked for others, worked long days, all while eating this way. So what I'm sharing isn't theory. It's real life.

You're not going to find fancy food here. I don't believe in using obscure ingredients that cost a fortune or leave you guessing. I'm not here to make things complicated. If you've got a fork, a pan, and the ability to avoid mixing the wrong foods on your plate, you're good to go.

You'll learn the basics. What to eat together. What to keep apart. When to eat fruit. How to structure your day. There are charts, sample meals, and recipes that actually make sense. I've even added some thoughts on Asian cooking, since that's part of how I eat too.

If you've struggled with bloating, slow digestion, weight gain, or just feeling off after eating, I'm telling you, this can change everything. But you've got to give it a proper go. Not for three days. Try it for three months, like I did. You'll see.

This isn't a diet you survive for a few weeks. It's something you can live with.

Let's get into it.

Chapter 1: The Wake up Call!

Before I talk about what this way of eating actually is, let me tell you why I started it in the first place. Because it wasn't some planned health kick. I didn't find this diet in a clinic. I wasn't handed a personalised nutrition plan by some expert. I found it out of desperation, because nothing else was working.

My wife was unwell. She had a hiatus hernia, and it flared up badly one evening after a heavy meal. I still remember that night vividly. We'd eaten out, something spicy, rich, and full of the usual suspects. Within hours, she was in pain. Not just discomfort or bloating, but that kind of sickness where your whole body rejects what you've eaten. Watching her go through that was frightening. It made me realise just how fragile our bodies can be when we keep feeding them things they were never designed to handle together.

That moment sparked something in me. I was carrying more weight than I liked, 190 pounds at the time, and I had grown used to feeling tired after meals. Heavy. Bloated. Sometimes my gut would make these strange noises for hours, like it was still trying to process lunch by the time dinner arrived. I wasn't unwell in the medical sense, but I knew deep down that something was off. My food wasn't giving me energy; it was draining it.

So I made a decision. I decided to stop mixing the wrong foods together. That's all. No calorie counting, no portion measuring, no meal replacement shakes. I simply started being mindful of what I put on my plate at each meal. And within a few weeks, my entire body responded.

In 90 days, I dropped two stone. That's 28 pounds, gone. No dieting. No starving. I ate full meals. I just stopped forcing my digestion to fight battles it wasn't meant to fight. And the weight didn't come back. It's been 35 years, and I still weigh 162 pounds. Not because I've been obsessive or lucky, but because my body found its balance and stayed there.

What's more important than the weight, though, is what changed on the inside. The tiredness faded. The bloating disappeared. My skin looked clearer. My head felt lighter. I stopped waking up with aches. My energy stopped crashing in the middle of the day. I started feeling like my body was working with me, not against me.

That early phase wasn't all easy. The first week or so, I felt rough. And I won't lie about it. When you've been eating a certain way for years, your body gets used to it, even if that way is damaging. So when I stopped mixing proteins and carbs together, when I gave my system a break, it had to clean house. That meant some headaches, some fatigue, and a lot more time in the bathroom. But that wasn't a sign to stop. It was a sign that my body was finally clearing out what it had been holding onto for too long.

Now, I go to the toilet three or four times a day. That might sound strange to some people, especially if you're used to thinking once a day, or every other day, is normal. But when your digestion works the way it's meant to, you eliminate waste easily and often. There's no straining, no discomfort, no bloated pressure in your gut. It just works. And you feel the difference in every part of your life.

This wasn't a miracle. It was a correction. A change back to eating in a way that makes sense for the body. Nothing extreme. Nothing complicated. Just choosing to build each meal properly, and letting the body do the rest.

That's where this journey began. Not with a diet plan, not with a goal weight, but with a question that's guided me ever since:

Am I worth it?

Because once you ask that seriously, and answer it with action, everything starts to change. This isn't a trend. It's not a diet that comes with branded snacks or subscription plans. The Hay Diet works because it follows how your body actually digests food. Once you understand that, everything else starts to make sense.

So what is the Hay Diet?

Let me clear up something straight away. This diet isn't about cutting things out or starving yourself. It's not a list of forbidden foods and green smoothies. It doesn't care about calorie counting or how many steps you walked today.

Instead, the Hay Diet focuses on **food combining**, learning which foods go together, and which don't. That's the heart of it. You still eat real food. You still eat three full meals a day. You don't skip anything, and you don't live on lettuce. All you change is *how* your meals are built.

Instead of throwing proteins and carbohydrates together on the same plate, like steak and chips or eggs and toast, you start learning which foods your stomach can actually digest together. You pair the right foods in a way that supports your digestion, instead of fighting it.

That's it.

It might sound too simple to matter, but that one change has changed my entire life. And not just mine. I've seen this help other people too, with their weight, their sleep, their moods, their digestion, their skin, even their mental clarity.

What Your Body's Been Trying to Tell You

Most people spend years trying to improve their health by focusing on the wrong things. They join gyms, track steps, cut down calories, and skip meals, yet still feel sluggish, heavy, or unwell. What they rarely consider is that the way their food is combined might be working against their body, meal after meal.

Your stomach has rules. It uses different enzymes and pH levels to break down protein, carbs, and fats. When you throw everything onto one plate, you're forcing your body to fight itself. That's what leads to the sluggishness, the acid, the gas, the bloating. You're not broken. You're just mixing foods that were never meant to be combined.

Your body is built to process different types of food under specific conditions. Proteins and carbohydrates, for example, require opposite environments for digestion. Protein needs an acidic setting with enzymes that break it down slowly and thoroughly. Carbohydrates, on the other hand, need an alkaline setting and work best when they pass through the stomach quickly. If you combine both in the same meal, your body can't handle them efficiently. The result is bad digestion.

I didn't realise it at first. Like everyone else, I thought eating "balanced meals" meant mixing everything together on one plate. Meat and potatoes. Eggs on toast. Fish with chips. But once I stopped doing that, once I gave my digestion a clear path to follow, I noticed how differently my body responded. I didn't just lose weight, I felt lighter, more focused, and more at ease after meals. There was no heaviness, no discomfort, and no sudden urge to lie down after eating.

The truth is, your body is constantly rebuilding itself. Every cell you have today is on its way to being replaced. Over a seven to nine-year cycle, your system renews itself piece by piece, it's not just my personal belief, it's a fact backed by several studies. That means the choices you make today don't just affect your current energy or digestion, they directly shape the body you're going to live in for the next decade. And if that rebuilding happens while your digestion is calm, steady, and efficient, you will feel it across every part of your health.

This way of eating doesn't just manage symptoms. It supports the systems that keep you alive and well. When your digestion runs smoothly, your immune function improves. Your skin becomes clearer. Your energy doesn't crash mid-afternoon. You sleep better. You move better. And you start recognising what your body actually needs, instead of reacting to cravings or habits that were never helping you in the first place.

This is the foundation of the Hay Diet. It does not ask you to remove entire food groups or give up the things you enjoy. It only asks you to stop putting the wrong ones together. Once you understand which foods work well in combination, and which ones clash, the process becomes simple. It's not a short-term diet. It's a quiet correction that stays with you.

You'll begin to recognise when a meal is working for you and when it isn't. You'll know when to stop, when to wait, and when to adjust, not because a chart told you to, but because your body finally has the space to respond with clarity.

That's what proper food combining offers. Not a trick. Not a trend. A cleaner path for your body to do what it was built to do.

A Way of Living, Not a Diet

Most diets feel like punishment. They tell you what you're not allowed to eat, how much is too much, and leave you feeling like you're constantly trying to earn your next meal. You're either "on" the plan or "off" it. And as soon as life gets in the way, when you're tired, travelling, busy, or just fed up, it's easy to fall back into old habits, not because you've failed, but because the system was never built for real life.

That's why I've never called this a diet. Not in the way people usually mean it.

This is a way of eating that fits into your day. It doesn't rely on willpower or strict measurements. It works because it makes sense. You're not forcing your body into submission, you're working with how it's already designed. Once you understand what to combine, the rest falls into place. You start choosing meals that help your body function instead of confusing it.

You won't need to weigh your food or scan every label like a detective. You won't have to eat separate meals from the rest of your family. You'll eat real food, just matched the right way. The only rule is: don't mix what clashes. That alone is enough to reset your digestion and take pressure off your system.

And when you're not overloaded, your body can handle life better. That includes the days you miss a meal, or the ones when you're out with friends and the options aren't ideal. You'll learn how to make better choices without becoming obsessive. If you get it wrong one day, you won't panic. You'll know how to come back to balance the next day, no guilt, no spiral.

That's the difference. When food combining becomes normal, you're no longer counting down to your next cheat day. You don't need one. There's no "off" switch. You're just eating well, most of the time, and your body thanks you for it.

And here's what most people don't expect: your cravings begin to change. When your digestion is calm, and your blood sugar isn't being pulled in every direction, you won't reach for snacks out of habit. You'll feel full from your meals, not stuffed and still unsatisfied. That constant search for something sweet, salty, or heavy after meals will also begin to fade.

This isn't wishful thinking. I've lived it. I've eaten like this through travel, birthdays, holidays, and everyday life. It hasn't restricted me. It's freed me. There's something powerful about knowing you can enjoy a proper meal without feeling tired afterwards, without feeling bloated for hours, without having to lie down just to cope with what you've eaten.

And when you build this way of eating into your routine, your health begins to hold steady. No constant swinging back and forth. No yo-yo weight changes. No seasonal health crashes.

Just stability. That's what this gives you, not temporary results, but a foundation you can keep going without effort.

So before we move into how the Hay Diet actually works, the categories, the charts, the combinations, pause here. Because this isn't a health hack. It's a return to common sense. It's the moment when eating becomes simple again, and your body finally gets a chance to function without confusion.

Once you experience that, you won't want to go back. Not because someone told you not to, but because your body will make it clear, in the best way possible.

Chapter 2: Understanding Food Combining

Most people never stop to question what happens after they eat. They're focused on how much they're eating, or whether it's "healthy" or "clean," but they don't think about what happens once it's inside their stomach. That's where everything really begins, and where most of the damage happens too.

I'm not saying that what you eat isn't important, it is! But how you combine those foods at each meal is where everything either works or falls apart. And that's exactly what we'll cover in this chapter.

You see, this way of eating is very simple. You don't need to give up real food. You don't need to count anything. You just need to stop throwing the wrong things together on the same plate. Once you do that, your digestion finally has a chance to catch its breath. You stop feeling bloated. You stop needing to lie down after lunch. You feel lighter, not because you've eaten less, but because your gut isn't under pressure.

Basically this is what food combining all about, learning which foods work well together and which don't. It means understanding what your body can handle at one time. Once you start doing that, you'll notice a difference very quickly, less gas, better bowel movements, clearer thinking, fewer crashes after eating.

Now in this chapter, I will walk you through the three food groups that matter here, protein, carbohydrate, and neutral, and how to combine them properly. It's not complicated. Once you get the hang of it, it becomes second nature. You'll look at a plate of food and know straight away whether it'll leave you feeling good or heavy and tired.

That's all food combining is. Not rules for the sake of rules. Just giving your body a proper chance to work with what you're eating, instead of having to clean up after it.

The Basics of Food Combining

When most people think about improving their diet, they think about what foods they need to eat more of, or which ones they should cut out completely. But what they usually miss is something much simpler, and more powerful. It's not just what you eat. It's how you combine it.

This way of eating starts with one basic idea: every food you put on your plate falls into one of three categories. Once you understand these categories, you'll be able to build meals that help your digestion instead of blocking it.

I am not talking about the food pyramid or calorie charts. This is much more practical. Every meal you eat should start with one of the following:

- **Protein foods:** This includes meat, fish, eggs, cheese, natural yogurt, tofu, and nuts. These foods need a strong acidic environment in the stomach to break down properly. Protein takes longer to digest and needs more effort from your system, which is fine, if it's not being forced to share space with something that works against it.

- **Carbohydrate foods:** these are your starches and grains. For example, bread, rice, pasta, oats, potatoes and legumes. They need a mildly alkaline environment to digest well. Your body uses a different set of enzymes here, and if acid is present, those enzymes get blocked.

- **Neutral foods:** These are your vegetables (except starchy ones like potatoes), leafy greens, herbs, salad, olive oil, avocado, lemon, and unsweetened non-dairy milk. They don't cause conflict in digestion and can be combined with either protein or carbohydrate meals without a problem. They help keep things moving and prevent the system from getting backed up.

That's it. Those are the three. The main principle of food combining is not to combine proteins and carbohydrates in the same meal.

By now you must be thinking, why does that even matter? Why can't I just eat a sandwich like everyone else?

Let me answer that now. You see that is because proteins and carbohydrates need completely different conditions to digest. Your stomach isn't a blender. It doesn't just mash everything up and send it down the line. It's a chemical system. And each type of food sets off a different process.

That's not opinion, that's basic human biology.

For example, when you eat protein, say, a piece of chicken or an egg, your stomach has to produce a strong acid and release specific enzymes to break it down. This process is slow, but necessary.

Now if you eat carbohydrates at the same time, like bread, rice, or pasta, your stomach is being asked to do the opposite. Carbs need a more alkaline environment, and they move through the system much faster.

You've now got two very different tasks happening in the same space, at the same time. One food group wants to slow down and be digested in acid. The other wants to move quickly through a gentler, alkaline setting. Your stomach can't do both at once.

What ends up happening is conflict. Your body tries to respond, but it's being asked to run two opposing systems at the same time. The acid for the protein blocks the enzymes for the starch. The whole thing slows down. Food lingers. It turns sour in your gut before it can be broken down. That's not digestion. That's fermentation.

If this happens once in a while, your body will cope. But most people eat like this three times a day, every day. Breakfast: toast and eggs. Lunch: sandwich with meat and bread. Dinner: pasta with chicken or steak with potatoes. It never gets a break.

The digestive system is constantly in damage control, trying to process food that was never meant to be digested together.

That's where the discomfort comes from. Not the amount of food. Not even the type. Just the combination.

When you stop putting these conflicting foods on the same plate, your stomach finally has one clear job to do. The food moves through smoothly. You absorb more nutrients. You feel fuller without feeling stuffed. You go to the toilet more regularly, and with less effort. You're not carrying food around inside for hours waiting for your system to catch up.

This isn't a theory. It's what the digestive system was made for. And it's probably why you've felt better after some meals and worse after others, even when the ingredients seemed fine on their own.

Now that you know the reason behind keeping proteins and carbs apart, let's make it even clearer with real examples. This part usually surprises people, because it includes so many of the meals we've been taught to think of as normal or even healthy.

Good and Bad Combinations

Let's start with some of the most common food combinations that cause problems:

- Eggs on toast, sounds like a good breakfast, but it's a protein and a starch in one bite. Your stomach can't break it down properly, and it leaves you feeling heavy or sluggish mid-morning.

- Steak and potatoes, both are whole foods, but the combination works against digestion. Steak needs acid and time. Potatoes need the opposite. The clash causes fermentation.

- Cheese sandwich, cheese is protein, bread is carb. The result is gas, discomfort, and poor absorption.

- Fish with chips or pasta with meat, the same principle. Too many meals like this and your gut starts to slow down over time.

Now compare those to meals that work with your digestion, not against it:

- Scrambled eggs with tomatoes and greens, all protein and neutral foods. Digests smoothly.

- Brown rice with stir-fried vegetables and olive oil, carbohydrate-based, with supportive neutrals. No conflict.

- Grilled chicken with spinach, cucumber, and avocado, a clean protein meal with neutral partners.

- Oats with banana and cinnamon, carb-based breakfast that doesn't confuse the system.

Each of these keeps one main group as the focus, either protein or carbohydrate, and builds the rest of the plate using neutrals. That's how you take pressure off your stomach and still eat full, satisfying meals. You're not eating less. You're just combining smarter.

This approach doesn't take long to learn. After a few days of building meals this way, you'll be able to look at a plate and know whether it's going to digest well or not. You'll feel the difference after meals, and that feedback is what teaches you faster than any chart can.

Why This Works

You see, our stomach isn't just a pit where food sits until it disappears. It's a chemical environment. And the kind of environment it creates depends entirely on what you've eaten.

When you eat a piece of meat, for example, your body knows it needs to produce hydrochloric acid and a strong enzyme called pepsin to break that protein down. This process is slow and controlled. The food stays in the stomach for longer so it can be properly dismantled before it moves on.

When you eat something starchy, like rice or bread, your body responds differently. It produces alkaline enzymes in the mouth and small intestine, like amylase, to break down those carbohydrates. These foods are meant to move faster through the stomach, not hang around in acid.

Now put those two types of food on the same plate, and everything gets jammed.

The acid needed for protein shuts down the enzymes needed for carbohydrates. The carbs can't break down properly, so they start to ferment. Meanwhile, the protein isn't broken down fully either, so it stays in the gut longer than it should, often rotting or creating gas along the way.

You won't always feel this right away. Sometimes it shows up hours later, or as a pattern, constant tiredness after meals, irregular bowel movements, heaviness in the stomach, even skin breakouts. These are all signs that digestion is being compromised.

This isn't a new idea. In fact, studies have looked at this for years. Researchers found that when you eat proteins and carbohydrates together, digestion slows down because the stomach struggles to empty properly (Hunt & Stubbs, 1975). Another study looked at how enzymes behave when they're trying to break down tightly packed proteins. If the environment inside your gut isn't right, like when too many different foods are clashing, those enzymes can't work as they should (Fu, Akula, Thorpe, & Hellman, 2021).

But honestly, you don't need to read those studies to know something's wrong. You've probably felt it after a badly combined meal without even realising why.

I didn't share these studies to make you memorise the science. The only reason I shared them is to help you understand that there's a reason this method works. You're not just changing food habits for the sake of it. You're giving your body one clear job to do at each meal, so it can do it properly.

And when digestion improves, everything else starts to follow. Energy, mood, immunity, even skin, it all starts in the gut.

So now the question becomes: how do you build meals that work with your body instead of against it? What does that look like on a plate, day to day? That's where the chart comes in, and that's what we'll cover next.

Hay Diet Food Combining Chart

By this point, you've got the basics. You know your stomach needs clarity, not conflict. You know protein and carbohydrate shouldn't sit side by side on your plate. And you understand why so many common meals leave people bloated, tired, or running to the medicine cabinet.

But now you must be wondering, how do you use this in real life, without making it complicated?

This is where the food combining chart becomes useful. Not as something you need to memorise or follow like a rulebook, but as a reference point until this way of eating becomes second nature.

At every meal, you start with one decision: Will this be a protein-based meal, or a carbohydrate-based meal?

Once you've decided that, the rest is easy. You pair that main food group with as many neutral items as you like, things like leafy greens, vegetables, herbs, oils, and certain fruits that won't disrupt the digestive process.

You don't need fancy recipes. You don't need to measure or weigh anything. Just stick to one main group per meal, and keep it clean.

The chart on below shows which food types can and cannot be combined in the same meal.

Hay diet food combining chart

Proteins and Carbohydrates are not compatible and shouldn't be used together.

Neutral foods can be combined with both.

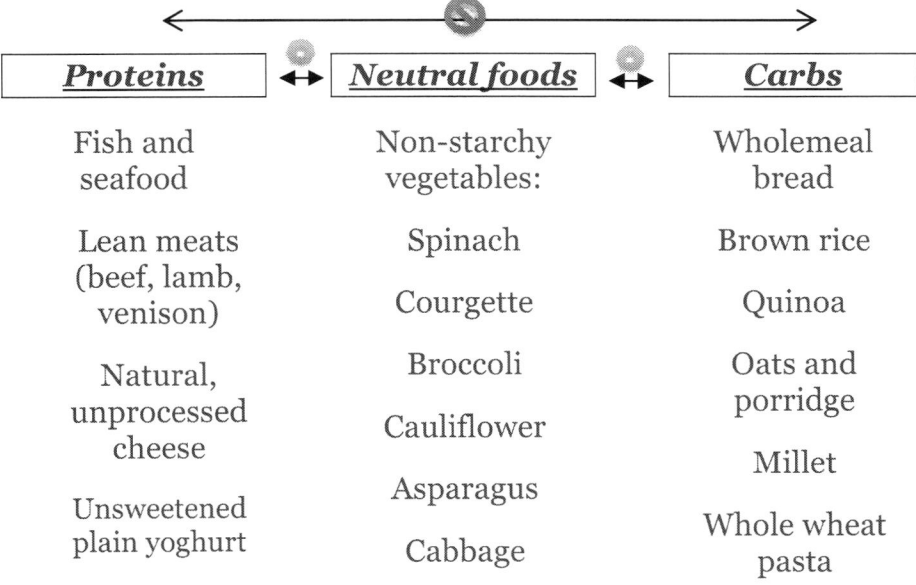

Proteins	Neutral foods	Carbs
Fish and seafood	Non-starchy vegetables:	Wholemeal bread
Lean meats (beef, lamb, venison)	Spinach	Brown rice
	Courgette	Quinoa
Natural, unprocessed cheese	Broccoli	Oats and porridge
	Cauliflower	Millet
Unsweetened plain yoghurt	Asparagus	Whole wheat pasta
	Cabbage	

Tofu and soy products

Nuts and seeds (in small amounts only)

Kale

Pak choi

Aubergine

Mushrooms

Peppers (bell)

Tomatoes (small quantities)

Cucumber

Lettuce and salad greens

Celery

Fennel

Avocados

Olives

Natural oils (olive oil, coconut oil, sesame oil)

Herbs and spices

Lemon or lime juice

Vinegar (apple cider, white wine, etc.)

Potatoes (white or sweet)

Corn and sweetcorn

Lentils

Chickpeas

Beans (e.g. kidney beans, black beans, counted here, not as protein)

Chapter 3: Gut Health and Regularity

Let's be honest, nobody really talks about what happens in the toilet. But I will. Because if your bowels aren't working properly, no amount of good food, supplements, or motivation is going to save you. The uncomfortable, bloated, stuck feeling most people have after a meal, that's not normal. It's a sign something's off in your gut. And if you're only going to the toilet once every couple of days, trust me, that's not regular. That's delayed.

Now I don't mean to sound blunt, but I've been on the Hay Diet for 35 years and I go to the toilet three to four times a day. Not once. Not every other day. Three to four. That's what proper digestion looks like. That's what happens when your meals move through you smoothly, without clashing and fermenting inside you like some slow, backed-up traffic jam.

You're supposed to eat food, digest it, and get rid of what your body doesn't need, not let it sit in your gut for half the day. And when you eat the wrong combinations, like eggs and toast or meat and potatoes, it slows the whole system down. Your stomach gets confused. Your bowels get lazy. And that's when the problems start.

Bloating. Gas. Constipation. That heavy, uncomfortable pressure in your belly that won't go away.

People often ask me, "How do I know if my gut's working right?" And I tell them: check your stools. Seriously. What comes out of you tells the truth about what's going on inside. Your stools should be soft, brown, and easy to pass. Not black, not dry, not hard. You shouldn't be straining. You shouldn't feel like you've only half gone. You shouldn't need ten minutes and a prayer just to feel relief.

The Hay Diet gets you back in rhythm with nature. It doesn't just clean up your plate, it cleans up your gut. That's why I'm not just talking about weight loss or clearer skin or less heartburn. I'm talking about something so basic and overlooked: proper elimination. Going when you need to. Going fully. And feeling lighter after, not like you're still carrying the last two meals around with you.

When Digestion Slows, Everything Suffers

Most people don't realise just how much their gut affects the rest of their life. If your bowels are sluggish, you'll feel it everywhere. In your mood. In your joints. In your sleep. You'll carry this vague discomfort around, a tight waistline, a foggy head, that sense of heaviness after eating that makes you want to lie down instead of live.

And the worst part is that most people think it's normal.

They think it's just part of ageing. Or that they need more fibre. Or more pills. Or that maybe they're just sensitive to everything now. But in my experience, it's not the food, it's the way it's being mixed. You eat chicken and chips, then wonder why your stomach feels like a brick. You start your day with toast and eggs and wonder why you're bloated by 10 a.m.

It's not a mystery. It's bad combinations sitting too long in the gut.

When you combine proteins and carbs in the same meal, your stomach has to pick a side. It can't fully digest both at once. So instead of breaking food down cleanly, it slows, stalls, and starts to ferment. That's what causes the gas, the trapped wind, the acid, the reflux, and the bloating. Now, speaking of bloating, many people often associate it with fat. The first thought that comes to their mind is that: "Maybe I'm bloated because the of the fat in my diet". But I want you to understand that it can be fat once. But if it happens in a routine and especially after everything you eat, that's not fat. It's food that hasn't moved.

I've spoken to people who've gone years thinking they were allergic to half the foods on their plate, when really, they were just combining them wrong. Once they followed the Hay Diet properly, keeping proteins and carbs in separate meals, eating vegetables with everything, staying hydrated, it was like someone flipped a switch in their gut. Things inside started moving again. Comfort came back. Even their skin looked better.

That's the power of proper digestion. It doesn't just make you feel lighter; it clears out the internal backlog you've probably forgotten was even there.

And honestly, you don't need a fancy test to tell you if your gut's healthy. Your body will show you. Every single day. And once you've been on this diet for a few days, you'll start noticing the difference, not just in the bathroom, but in how you feel after every meal.

Nonetheless, just to give you an idea, this is what a well-functioning gut actually looks like:

- You go to the toilet at least once or twice a day, and I mean fully. No stopping and starting. No effort.

- You feel light after meals, not heavy or swollen.

- Your stomach doesn't make strange noises for hours after eating.

- There's no urge to unbutton your trousers at the table.

- You stop getting that trapped wind or the strange bubbling that makes you wonder if something's wrong.

- You don't carry that sluggish, bloated feeling from morning until night.

- And most important, your bowel movements become soft, brown, and natural. Like your body's doing what it was meant to do.

I know it might sound strange to focus a whole chapter on toilet habits, but this is where most people get it wrong. They ignore the signals. They assume irregularity is just "their normal." But once they actually experience a clean, consistent digestive rhythm, they realise how far off track they were before.

Your gut should not feel like a guessing game.

It's supposed to feel calm. Predictable. Balanced.

That's what the Hay Diet restores.

Because when you stop mixing food in ways your body can't handle, everything starts to move again. Not in a violent, laxative kind of way (We all know that's actually worse than being bloated). But in a natural, consistent, comfortable flow. Like you've taken the brakes off your own system, and finally let it work the way it was meant to.

Now you might be thinking, "Isn't this just a high-fibre diet in disguise?" And no, it's not. Fibre helps, of course. But fibre alone won't fix your gut if your food is still clashing in your stomach like a traffic accident.

Why Fibre Alone Isn't Enough

You can pile on all the veg and oats you want, but if you're still mixing steak with potatoes or eggs with toast, you'll keep running into the same problem, stuck digestion.

The issue isn't just what goes in; it's how it moves through your system.

The Hay Diet works because it takes pressure off your system. It lets each meal digest cleanly, with the enzymes and stomach conditions it needs. That's what makes the real difference. It's not about roughage. It's about flow.

Think of your stomach like a factory. If you send in two jobs that require totally different equipment, the whole line slows down. Nothing gets processed properly. That's what happens when you eat protein and starch together. One needs acid. One needs alkaline. Your body can't do both at the same time, so it stalls.

And when digestion stalls, waste builds up. You start feeling heavy. You stop going regularly. Your skin flares up. You get that cloudy head and short fuse. It's not just your bowels, it's your whole system backing up.

Fibre can't fix that if the food is still colliding. But once you clean up the combinations, that's when fibre starts working properly. That's when vegetables start moving things through. That's when hydration actually helps, instead of sloshing around in a gut that's locked up.

So no, this isn't just about adding fibre. It's about removing the chaos. Letting your meals work with your body, not against it.

That's when your gut breathes again. And trust me, you'll feel it.

The best part of it all is that once things start moving properly, they tend to stay that way, as long as you don't go back to the old food clashes. But over the years I have noticed that even with the right combinations, a few small habits make a huge difference in how smoothly things flow. There are a few habits (treat them more like a rule) that have been super helpful for me in the last 35 years. I have shared them below:

1. Eat Slowly. Chew Properly.
This sounds basic, but most people eat like they're on a timer. Chewing starts digestion, and if you rush it, your stomach has

to play catch-up. That's how undigested food ends up sitting around, causing problems.

2. Drink Water, but Not During Meals.
You want water, yes. But not while you're eating. Sipping with meals waters down your stomach acid. That slows digestion. So drink between meals. A glass first thing in the morning is a great start. Warm water with lemon helps too.

3. No Dessert After Lunch or Dinner.
This one is very important. When you eat fruit or sweets after a full meal, they ferment. You might not notice it immediately, but that sudden bloated feeling you get an hour later is dessert turning to gas. Keep fruit between meals, at least an hour before or two hours after.

4. Stick to the Combining Rules, Even When You're Tired.
Some days you won't feel like cooking. That's fine. Keep some basics ingredients ready, like boiled eggs (for protein meals), cooked brown rice (for carb meals), and chopped veggies (which work with both), so you can throw together a proper meal without overthinking it. Just make sure not to mix proteins and crabs.

5. Don't Mix for the Sake of Flavour.
A lot of people throw everything on one plate because it "tastes good." But you'd be amazed to know that when your digestion is smooth and your gut feels clean, you stop craving complicated plates. You start to prefer the way simple meals make you feel, light, steady, and pain-free.

Now, I'm not saying that you have to be perfect at these, but my advice is to at least try to maintain a steady rhythm. Once you've got it, you'll know. And once your gut gets into that daily flow, you'll realise it was dragging everything else down with it.

By everything, I don't just mean going to the toilet more often, I'm talking about what happens after you do. That lightness you feel, the clarity, and the sudden calm in your body. These are not just in your head. It's what real digestion feels like.

I've had people tell me their skin cleared up within weeks. Others say their migraines eased. I can't count how many said they suddenly had more patience with their family, less snappy, less foggy, just more present. That's not magic. That's a body that's not weighed down by internal chaos.

The Real Proof Is in the Toilet

Look, you can weigh yourself. You can count calories. You can stare at labels all day. But none of that gives you real feedback the way your toilet does.

That's where the truth shows up.

You'll know the Hay Diet is working when you don't dread going to the bathroom anymore. When it doesn't feel like a battle or a waiting game. When you stop feeling like something's always "off" in your gut but you can't quite explain what.

That's what happened to me.

Three to four times a day. No discomfort. No pressure. Just clean, natural elimination. And that's been the case for decades now. Not just a good week or a few lucky days, it's become the baseline. Because once your gut gets used to working the way it was meant to, it doesn't need drama to do its job. It just works.

That's the kind of stability people don't talk about enough. You're not chasing results anymore; you're just living in them.

And it all starts with how you put food on your plate. Not how much. Not what time. Not which trend. Just how it's combined.

If there's one places your health will always leave clues, it's the toilet. So check in with your gut. It'll tell you more than any fitness tracker ever will.

And once you feel that daily rhythm return, trust me, you'll never want to go back.

Now, what might surprise you is just how much that change in your digestion starts to affect everything else. Your mood. Your clarity. Even how you handle stress.

Let's take a closer look at that in the next chapter.

Chapter 4: The Mind-Gut Connection

You can always tell when your stomach is upset, but what most people don't notice is how it messes with your mind too. You feel foggy. Moody. Drained. Like your brain is stuck in second gear and nothing feels sharp. You're not sick exactly... but you're definitely not yourself either.

I used to brush that off. I thought it was just age. Or stress. Or bad sleep. But the truth is, it was my gut. And when I started eating the Hay Diet way, combining my food properly, clearing out the backups, letting my digestion finally breathe, my mind started to come back online too.

That's not just my experience. It's something more and more people are waking up to. Researchers are finally confirming what people like me have been saying for years, the gut doesn't just handle food. It talks to your brain. All day long. And if that conversation is full of toxins, gas, and gut stress, you're going to feel it in your head, your mood, and your motivation.

So no, in this chapter we won't talk about digestion anymore. We already sorted that. Now we're getting into what happens after. When your gut starts healing, your mind starts clearing.

Let's start with the mind-gut connection.

The Second Brain, And It's Not in Your Head

They say your gut is your second brain. Honestly, I think for most people, it's the first. Because when your stomach's off, everything feels off. You wake up in a mood. You can't focus. You get irritated over nothing. You think it's stress or age or something in your head, but really, it's your digestion dragging everything down with it.

I didn't know any of this when I started. I just knew I felt foggy, tired, and heavy. My mind wasn't sharp. I wasn't sleeping properly. And I was getting snappy at things that normally wouldn't bother me. Once I got on the Hay Diet and sorted out what was happening in my gut, all of that started to ease. And I'm not just saying that. I felt it. In my head. In my mood. In how I handled the day.

Turns out your gut actually produces most of the feel-good stuff people think comes from the brain, like serotonin. Researchers call it the feel-good hormone. And when that area's clogged up or under strain, you don't just feel it in your stomach. You feel it in your mind too.

So when people ask me why they feel calmer on this diet, or why they're waking up with more energy or not feeling as anxious, this is why. It's not magic. It's not a mind-set hack. It's just that your gut's not sending the wrong signals to your brain anymore.

Once you stop putting food in that causes chaos, your system quiets down. The brain fog is gone and you feel steady again. Now, I have heard people say: how is that even possible. How can a simple diet fix brain-fog? You see, in most cases the real culprit behind brain fog is your gut.

How Food Combining Clears the Fog

Before I changed how I ate, I didn't even realise how foggy I'd become. I thought it was normal to feel wiped out after meals. Or to have a dip in the afternoon where I couldn't think clearly. Or to wake up already tired, like I hadn't rested at all.

It wasn't until I got off the bad combinations, eggs with toast, meat with potatoes, cheese on bread, that I noticed something change. Not just in my digestion, but in my head.

It's hard to explain unless you've felt it. You don't suddenly become a different person. You just stop dragging yourself through the day. You think clearer. You've got more patience. You don't feel like everything's ten times harder than it should be.

And it's not because of caffeine or supplements or positive thinking. It's because your gut isn't under pressure anymore. Your body's not using all its energy trying to untangle a plate full of mixed signals. When meals are simple and properly combined, digestion happens faster, smoother and the leftover heaviness completely disappears.

No bloating. No brain fog. No random crashes that hit you after lunch.

And the best part is, it happens naturally. No tracking. No obsessing. Just eat a clean diet, and your system thanks you by making everything feel lighter.

People always talk about mind-set first. "Get your head right, and your body will follow." But for me, it was the other way around.

Body First, Mind Follows

When I first started this diet, I wasn't trying to fix my mind. I wasn't reading about gut-brain connections or neurotransmitters or anything like that. I just wanted to stop feeling so awful all the time. My belly was a mess. My digestion was unpredictable. My energy was shot. I was fed up with blaming food, guessing what to cut out next, and still ending up with bloating or gas or just that miserable stuck feeling. So I changed how I combined my meals. That was it.

What came next, though, that was the surprise.

I'd been tired for years. Not exhausted, not sick, just constantly below baseline. I thought it was work. Or stress. Or getting older. But once I started eating this way, the tiredness lifted. Not in one magical moment. It just... faded. Day by day, I realised I wasn't dragging through the afternoon anymore. I wasn't waking up groggy. I wasn't losing track of what I was doing halfway through a task.

My head felt clearer. I could focus longer. I wasn't as reactive, I'd still get annoyed, sure, but it didn't stick. It passed. My mood wasn't bouncing all over the place. I wasn't on edge. I wasn't short-tempered for no reason. There was space between things. Breathing room.

I hadn't added anything fancy. No powders, no pills. I hadn't changed my job or taken time off or gone on some self-care trip. I'd just started putting different meals on my plate. I wasn't even trying to be "healthy" in the modern sense. I was just finally letting my gut do its job without interference.

And that changed everything.

You don't realise how loud your body's been until it finally quiets down. How much effort it takes to get through the day when your insides are in a constant state of tension. Once that pressure eases, when your gut is no longer jammed up, trying to process things it was never meant to handle together, it's like your whole system exhales. And your mind feels it first.

That's when I really understood the full picture. This wasn't just about digestion. This was about getting my balance back.

It's hard to describe unless you've lived it. But if you're reading this and nodding, because your patience is thin, your head's foggy, your mood flips for no reason, then please hear this: it might not be in your head. It might be in your gut.

And the moment your body starts working with you again, you'll feel it. In the silence. In the steadiness. In the fact that nothing feels as overwhelming anymore.

That's when you know it's working.

I didn't need a research paper to tell me any of this. I could feel it happening in my own body. But funnily enough, once I started looking into it years later, the science lined up exactly with what I'd already lived. And if you're the kind of person who wants more than just lived experience, if you want the studies and the facts to back it all up, then you're in luck. Because they're finally catching on.

Science and Hay Diet

Now, I'm not a scientist. Never claimed to be. But I pay attention. Especially when science starts backing up what I've been living for years.

When I first started this diet, nobody was talking about gut-brain anything. It was all calories, exercise, and portion sizes. Mental health did exist but it was a separate thing. But, now there's research everywhere connecting gut health to mood, clarity, even emotional resilience.

And honestly, I'm not surprised.

You don't need a lab coat to notice what happens when your digestion clears up. You just need to pay attention to your own body. The fog lifts, a steadiness creeps back in, these aren't mere coincidences. That's your gut doing less firefighting, and your brain finally getting some peace.

There's one study I came across recently that really stuck with me. It was published in *Social Science & Medicine* in 2020. They followed people through adolescence and tracked their fruit and vegetable intake. The more consistently people ate whole, plant-based foods, the better their mental health. Not just slightly better, clearly better. Less mood disruption, more focus, fewer signs of anxiety and low energy.

And that fits perfectly with what the Hay Diet is about. It's not some cleanse or restriction plan. It's real food, properly combined, with a focus on vegetables, hydration, and not mixing things that confuse your gut. That's what gets things flowing again. And once things flow, you start thinking clearer, sleeping deeper, coping better.

It doesn't mean life gets easier. It just means you're not wading through it half-asleep anymore.

When you stop throwing your digestion into chaos, protein and starch wrestling on the same plate, sugar mixed with fat, meals that sit heavy and take hours to move, your body settles. And when your body settles, your mind gets to rest too. It's all connected.

That's why when people say, "Oh, it's just food," I always think, no, it's not. It's never just food. It's how you feel after you eat. It's how you wake up the next morning. It's how quickly you snap at someone or how long you stay stuck in your own head. It's whether you can sit still and breathe properly or whether you're holding tension without even noticing.

That's not random. That's digestion. That's your gut talking.

And now the science is finally catching up to what so many of us have lived and felt all along. So if you've been feeling low, scattered, irritated, or mentally stuck, you're not sick. You're just overdue for a reset. And that reset starts in the gut.

The Symptoms Most People Miss

Most people think they'd know if their gut was off. They picture bloating, cramps, maybe a bit of constipation. But the truth is, it's rarely that obvious. For a lot of people, the signs are subtle. They show up in ways you don't even link to digestion, until you step back and really look.

For me, it wasn't just the physical discomfort. It was the tiredness that hung around no matter how early I went to bed. The short fuse I developed without even realising it. The way my brain just wouldn't stay on task. One minute I'd be focused, the next I'd forget what I'd even walked into the room for. It's easy to laugh that off, "Oh, I'm just getting older", but no. That wasn't age. That was my gut slowing everything down.

And I hear the same stories from other people who try the Hay Diet. They come into it hoping to lose weight or fix their digestion. They're not expecting their mind to clear up. They're not expecting their mood to level out. But it happens. Almost every time.

You'll hear things like:

- "I didn't realise how anxious I'd been until I wasn't anymore."
- "I used to feel overwhelmed all the time, now I can actually sit still and breathe."
- "I'm just not snapping like I used to, and it's not because life got easier."

That last one's important. Life doesn't have to change for your response to it to shift. Sometimes all it takes is sorting out your internal traffic jam, the one nobody talks about, the one that starts in the gut and ends up in your head.

You'd be amazed how many things we chalk up to personality, or stress, or hormones, that are really just symptoms of a system that hasn't been running properly. I've had people tell me their migraines eased. Their skin stopped breaking out. They're less jittery. Less reactive. More present. More themselves.

And it's not because they added something. It's because they stopped putting the wrong combinations in. No more meat and mash. No more cheese toasties. No more fish and chips, not because they're "bad foods," but because they clash in the gut and the whole system pays the price.

When you clear up the gut, these other symptoms, the ones you thought were just "how you are", start to lift.

So if you've been stuck in a cycle of fatigue, forgetfulness, low mood, or irritability, and you've tried everything else, maybe it's time to look lower. The answer might not be in your head at all. It might be right under your ribs, quietly asking for less chaos and more clarity.

The point I am trying to make is that once you start hay diet, sure, your digestions get better. But there's a point where you stop just feeling "better" physically, and you realise something deeper has changed. Your mind feels sharper. You feel calmer. You're no longer dragging yourself through the day. That's not from a supplement or a mind-set shift. That's what happens when your body finally stops working against itself.

And I didn't see it coming. I just wanted to stop feeling sluggish and uncomfortable after meals. But once I started eating the Hay Diet way, proper food combining, clean digestion, simple meals, the fog started to lift.

I could focus longer. I wasn't getting irritated over small things. I had more space in my head. That's the only way I can describe it. There was more room to think, to breathe, to just be present in my own life again.

It was like something heavy had been quietly pressing down on me for years, and I'd just accepted it. Then one day, it was gone.

Once the pressure inside me eased, my whole system caught up. I didn't need motivation or willpower. I just felt clearer. And the clearer I felt, the more I wanted to keep going.

And it's not just clarity, it's energy. Real, steady energy. Not bursts from caffeine or sugar. Just a sense that I had what I needed to handle the day.

"I wake up every day and I have NO aches or pains at all. I'm 66 years old. I feel 45."

That's the truth. No tension. No stiffness. No fog. I'm not chasing results; I've been living in them. And I'm not holding it together through strict habits or discipline. It's just what happens when the internal weight lifts and your body finally gets the space to do what it's meant to do.

That's what I want people to understand. This isn't just about digestion. This isn't just about food. This is about getting yourself back, the version of you that isn't constantly running on empty, reacting to everything, or feeling like you're two steps behind.

Once your system calms down, your thoughts calm down too. Your mood steadies. Your mind stops pushing through fog. And that emotional heaviness that used to follow you everywhere gets lighter.

That's why I've stayed on this diet. Not for the numbers on the scale, for this. The steadiness. The clarity. The feeling of actually being in my body again, without pain, without pressure, without that mental weight dragging behind me.

But there is also another benefit of eating this way. It's way better and more effective than traditional diets. It also helps you lose weight. Not because you're trying to lose it. But because your body's finally ready to let it go.

Let's talk more on the in the coming chapter.

Chapter 5: Natural Weight Loss Without Dieting

Most diets start with restriction. Less food. Less joy. Less of everything. You're told to cut back, weigh everything, obsess over numbers, feel guilty for eating anything that tastes good, and then somehow expect your body to respond with balance.

It never works. Not for long anyway.

That's the trap people fall into. They think losing weight means suffering. That if they're not hungry, they're doing it wrong. That if they're not counting every bite, they're slipping. And after a while, the whole thing just becomes one big mental weight, on top of the physical weight they were already carrying.

I've seen it over and over again. People push through diets for a few weeks, maybe a couple of months, and then crash. Not because they failed, but because the method was never built to last.

That's why the Hay Diet feels so different. It doesn't ask you to eat less. It doesn't tell you to cut out everything you love. You don't need a calculator. You don't need a scale. You don't need to be "perfect."

You just need to stop putting the wrong foods on the same plate.

That's it.

You're not starving yourself. You're not punishing your body. You're giving it a break. A proper one.

And that's what makes the weight start to move, not because you forced it, but because your system finally has the space to let go of what it's been holding onto.

This diet doesn't dictate what you can't have. It focuses more on *when* and *how* you have it. And once that clicks, the rest of it starts to make sense.

When I first started the Hay Diet, I wasn't even trying to lose weight. I just wanted to feel better. I was tired of feeling bloated, heavy, sluggish after meals, tired of guessing what food was "safe" and what was going to set things off. I didn't expect a transformation. I expected maybe a bit less discomfort.

But three months in, I stepped on the scale and I'd lost two stone.

"I went on the Hay Diet 35 years ago, when I weighed 190 lbs, and after I was on the diet for 90 days, I was 162 lbs. I'm still 162 lbs 35 years later."

I didn't exercise like mad. I didn't count calories. I didn't starve myself. I didn't cut out the foods I liked. I just stopped combining them in a way that confused my digestion.

That is when the transformation began.

For once, my body wasn't in panic mode after every meal. It wasn't trying to untangle a mix of protein and starch while also processing a bit of sugar, a few oils, and something acidic on top. It was just doing its job, cleanly, efficiently, without stress.

And because of that, my energy started coming back. My gut calmed down. The bloating went away. The water weight dropped. And the fat that was sitting around my middle and wouldn't budge no matter how little i eat, that started to melt too.

And I wasn't hungry.

That's the part most people can't believe. I was eating three proper meals a day. I felt full after every one. I wasn't snacking out of frustration. I wasn't waiting for the next meal like I was on a countdown clock. I just ate what worked, and my body responded in a way it never had before.

I didn't "lose weight." I just stopped holding onto it.

That's what happens when your digestion stops struggling, the body finally lets go of what it doesn't need.

And that weight has never come back.

Thirty-five years later, I'm still the same weight. Still eating three meals a day. Still not counting anything. Still not bouncing between diets. Just keeping my meals clean and separate, and letting my system do what it was meant to do.

Why Proper Combining Helps Burn Fat

Most people think weight loss comes from eating less. But they never stop to ask, less of *what*? They'll cut carbs, cut fat, cut everything but flavour and still feel bloated, still feel heavy. Still stuck.

It's not always the food itself. It's what happens when it lands in your stomach.

Take a plate of rice and fish. Or toast and eggs. On paper, nothing wrong with either. But when you eat them together, your body doesn't know what job to do first. Protein needs one type of digestive environment. Carbs need another. And when both show up at once, things start to clash.

Your stomach stalls. Digestion slows. The food sits longer than it should. And instead of giving you energy, it starts to ferment, not in a good way. That's what leads to bloating, pressure, gas, water weight. Your metabolism isn't broken; it's just bogged down.

Now change the combinations, keep protein meals and carb meals separate, and pair them with neutral vegetables. Suddenly, digestion becomes simple. The gut works through it without strain. Digesting one food at a time. No conflict. No backup.

That's when things start to change.

Your body stops wasting energy on fighting food combinations and starts using that energy for what it's meant to do, breaking down nutrients, absorbing what you need, and letting go of the rest.

And that includes fat.

When your gut is calm and meals digest cleanly, your system isn't bloated or waterlogged. Your metabolism isn't confused. You're not sending mixed signals. You're feeding it in a way that works, and the weight starts to move.

Not because you've restricted anything. But because your body isn't being slowed down by chaos every time you eat.

That's what proper food combining does. It creates clarity, inside and out.

You're Not Bloated, You're Stalled

A lot of people look in the mirror and think they're gaining fat. But half the time, it's not fat at all, it's bloat. It's water. It's food that hasn't moved properly. It's meals that are still sitting inside you, hours after you've finished eating.

And the worst part is, they blame themselves. They think they're not trying hard enough. So they start eating less. Skipping meals. Cutting down even more, and still, nothing changes. The heaviness stays. The trousers feel tight. The scale won't move. Because the issue isn't how much they're eating. It's how their body is dealing with it.

Once I understood that, everything changed.

When I stopped mixing conflicting foods, protein and starch on the same plate, sugar with fat, acid with dairy, my stomach stopped swelling after meals. I wasn't walking around with that "full but still hungry" feeling. I didn't need to lie down after eating. I didn't feel like I had to unbuckle my belt after lunch.

That wasn't fat. That was digestive traffic.

And when the traffic clears, your body starts letting go. Of the bloating. Of the water retention. Of the backup that's been sitting there for days, sometimes weeks. And that's when real fat loss becomes possible, not because you're restricting, but because your body's not stuck anymore.

Most people are carrying weight that isn't even theirs to carry. It's leftover meals that didn't move. It's swelling from constant food stress. It's inflammation from bad combinations.

But once you start combining foods the right way, your gut stops fighting. Meals pass through. Your stomach stays flat. You don't feel stuffed all the time. You don't feel swollen or blocked or like something's always "off."

You just feel normal. And after years of bloating and discomfort, *normal* feels incredible.

That's when you realise, you weren't gaining weight. You were just never clearing it.

You Eat What You Like, Just Not All Together

The thing people always ask is, "But do I have to give up my favourite foods?"

And the answer is no. Not unless your favourite food is a cheeseburger with chips, eaten in one go. Because it's not about cutting things out, it's about separating them. That's all.

You don't need to ditch bread. Or meat. Or cheese. You just don't eat them all on the same plate. You don't mix protein with starch, or fruit with a full meal. You don't follow up lunch with dessert, or eat toast and eggs together just because it's what you grew up on.

46

Once you know how your digestion works, you start building meals that support it, not confuse it.

And the best part is: you're not hungry.

You're eating proper meals. Real food. Not grazing all day, not counting anything, not walking around thinking about your next snack. When you eat food that digests cleanly, you actually stay full. Your body knows what to do with it, and it moves on.

There's no guilt around portion size. No weighing. No tracking. You eat what you like, just not all at once.

"You will be slim, fit, happy, optimistic, fun, all these things will be possible when you do this diet."

I believe that. Because that's what happened to me.

I didn't lose weight because I followed some perfect routine or became ultra-disciplined. I just stopped confusing my system. I didn't try to eat less. I just gave my body space to process what I was eating. The meals were still satisfying. They still had flavour. I didn't feel like I was missing out.

It's not about sacrifice. It's about structure. That's what makes it liveable. That's what makes it stick.

And once it clicks, you stop thinking about food all the time, because your body's not screaming for attention after every bite.

I didn't need a study to tell me this worked. I'd already seen it. I felt lighter. My digestion was smoother. The weight dropped and stayed off. But years later, I came across a bit of research that made me smile, not because it taught me something new, but because it confirmed what I'd been doing all along.

The *Journal of the American Medical Association* published a study in 2012 that tracked people who had already lost weight. The question was: how do you keep it off long-term? What they found was interesting, it wasn't just about calories. It was about how meals were structured. The composition of your food, and the effect that has on hormones and metabolism, mattered more than the calorie count.

That's exactly what this diet is built on.

When you eat meals your body can process efficiently, meals that aren't clashing or causing internal stress, you use energy better. You stay full longer. Your system isn't stuck in clean-up mode all the time. So it holds onto less.

They used complicated words in the study, of course, metabolic adaptation, energy expenditure, glycaemic load. But I didn't need any of that to know the basics: when meals are simple and properly combined, your body responds.

You don't overeat because you don't need to. You don't get weird hunger spikes or sugar crashes. Your gut stays calm. Your energy stays steady. And your body lets go of what it no longer needs, including weight.

This isn't just my theory. It's just what happens when you stop forcing your digestion to wrestle with your plate.

The funny thing is, once your meals start digesting properly, you stop thinking about food all the time. You're not obsessing. You're not clock-watching. You're not counting the hours until the next thing. You just feel steady.

That's what people don't expect. They think they'll have to work hard to stop overeating. They think they need more discipline, more self-control. But when your gut isn't confused and bloated and inflamed, your hunger signals calm down too. You eat when you're actually hungry. You stop when you're full. And that's it.

Before this diet, I was always chasing food. Not because I was greedy, but because I never felt properly satisfied. I'd eat a meal, and half an hour later I'd feel like I needed something else. Or I'd be completely full, but still poking around for something sweet. It was all over the place.

That doesn't happen anymore.

Now, I eat three proper meals a day, clean, well-combined, no clutter, and I don't even think about food between them. I'm not forcing anything. I'm not restricting myself. I'm just not hungry all the time.

That's the part that surprises people the most. You don't stop overeating because of willpower. You stop because your body isn't sending you confused messages anymore.

Once your system is running clearly, your appetite finds its own rhythm. No tracking, no guilt, no tricks. Just a body that's finally working the way it should.

But before all that settles in, before you find your rhythm, there's something else that usually happens first. Your body has to clear out what's already inside. And I'll be honest, those first few days can feel quite rough.

Let's talk about that next.

Chapter 6: Detox and Body Reset

Let's get one thing clear, this isn't some juice cleanse or five-day fast where you starve yourself on celery water and call it a reboot. That's not what the Hay Diet is about. But make no mistake, your body *will* detox when you start this way of eating. Not because you're forcing it, but because you're finally stepping out of its way.

For years, most of us have eaten in a way that clogs up our system, mixing things that were never meant to digest together. Meat and potatoes, eggs and toast, fish and rice. It's not that these foods are bad. It's how we throw them all into one meal and expect the body to just deal with it. That's where the trouble begins. Fermentation, gas, bloating, sluggish bowels, all of it builds up quietly, day after day. And you get used to it. That heavy, bloated feeling becomes normal.

Then you switch to the Hay Diet. You stop mixing protein and carbs. You simplify your meals. And just like that, your gut starts working properly again. That's when the real clean-up begins.

That's not me being dramatic. That's the truth.

You might get headaches. You might feel bloated. You might be unusually tired. Your skin might look a bit worse before it improves. Some people even feel a bit low, like their mood takes a dip before it starts to rise again.

This isn't because the diet is doing something wrong. It's because it's finally doing something right. Your body's clearing the leftovers, not just the food sitting in your gut, but all the stuff it hasn't had time to properly deal with for years.

When you stop sending in food that clashes, and you finally let your stomach do one job at a time, your system starts clearing the mess. That takes energy. It takes work. And for a few days, you might feel like it's all going backwards.

That's normal.

It's not a sign to quit. It's a sign that something's finally happening. For the first time in years, your body isn't drowning in new chaos, it's catching up on old damage. And yes, it feels uncomfortable. But that's part of the reset. You don't get clean without moving some dirt first.

Give it a week. Just one. Most people feel the lift around day eight. Some sooner. But by then, you'll know it was worth sticking with.

What's Actually Happening in the First Week

You know how people say, "It gets worse before it gets better"? That's exactly what happens here. Not because the Hay Diet is harsh, it's not. But because your body's been stuck in clean-up mode for years without a break, and now it finally has a chance to do its job properly.

So, what happens in that first stretch?

Let's talk about it like it is.

You might get a headache. Nothing dramatic, just this dull, nagging weight in your head, especially if you've been living on caffeine, sugar, or processed snacks. Your body's not getting its usual chemical hits, and it doesn't know what to do with the silence. That's withdrawal. Not from food, but from the stuff hidden *in* the food.

You might feel a bit off, slower than usual, like your energy's in low gear. Your gut is busy clearing out the mess. That takes real energy. It's not the time for HIIT workouts or running marathons. It's the time to let your system breathe.

Your toilet habits will probably change. And trust me, that's a good thing. You'll likely start going more often, two, maybe three times a day. And when you go, it'll feel easier. Your stools won't be hard or dry. They'll be soft, brown, and clean. That's a clear sign your digestion is waking up.

You might feel bloated, weirdly enough. Not the same bloating as before, but this internal shifting, like your system's moving things out. And yes, there might be some gas. Don't panic. It's not forever. It's just your body reacting to finally being fed food it can process properly.

One more thing: your cravings might go wild. Not because you're hungry, but because your old habits are flaring up. The need to snack, to grab something sweet after dinner, that's your old routine dying off. If you can ride that wave, it passes. And when it does, it feels like freedom.

I've been through all of this. And I've watched others go through it too. The ones who hang in there, past the first 7–10 days, start to feel different. Lighter, not just in their body but in their mood. Calmer. More focused. Less reactive.

That's when you'll know, it's working.

So if you're on day three or four and thinking, "Is this worth it?" I want you to keep going. It's your body finally doing what it hasn't been able to do for far too long.

How to Support the Detox (Without Getting Extreme)

Now that you know what's coming, let's talk about how to make it easier. You don't have to just sit there and suffer through the first 7 to 10 days. There's plenty you can do to help your body along without making things worse. I have shared a few tips below:

Get your vegetables in, and blend them if you need to.

Raw veg helps clean out the gut, but if your stomach is already touchy, it can feel like too much. A blender makes that easier.

You might be better to buy or use your blender, to eat some of your vegetables raw. This has been found to reduce the acid in your stomach to acceptable levels.

Even a mix of cucumber, spinach, and celery with a bit of lemon can help your system start clearing without much effort. It's light, it digests quickly, and it gives your stomach a break.

Drink water, but not with food.

You need water now more than ever, but gulping it down during meals just waters everything out. That slows digestion. It's better to drink between meals, especially early in the day and in the late afternoon. You'll feel the difference when your body isn't bogged down trying to digest and flush at the same time.

Cut the white flour and sugar.

White bread, biscuits, pasta, fizzy drinks, they all add to the backup. When you remove them, things change fast. Your gut stops swelling, your breath improves, and you stop feeling like food's still sitting with you long after you've eaten. Your body doesn't want these things. It's just used to them.

Use clean fats and keep the meals light.

Stick to olive oil, avocado, a small handful of soaked seeds, just enough to support digestion. Skip the heavy sauces and deep frying. Meals don't need to be complicated or rich to work. Right now, the goal is to give your body less to clean up, not more.

Keep meals simple.

Pick one core food, either protein or carbs, and build the meal around that. Add vegetables, and let that be enough. You're not trying to impress anyone. You're just helping your body reset, without overwhelming it again. This is when neutral combinations really shine. They get the job done quietly.

You don't need to do more. You just need to give your system a clear path and let it get on with the detox it's been trying to do for years. Which It will, if you stop getting in the way.

People hear the word detox and think of green juices, powders, skipping meals, or some harsh plan you can only survive for a few days. But when the food you eat actually supports your digestion, and doesn't fight it, your body detoxes on its own.

That's what proper food combining does. It takes away the internal traffic jams that cause everything to slow down, the bloating, the gas, the bad breath, the heaviness after meals. Those aren't just uncomfortable side effects. They're signs your system is backed up. When you stop throwing conflicting signals at your stomach, your body gets the space it needs to clean up.

This isn't something you force. It happens on its own. When digestion works the way it should, waste doesn't sit around fermenting. Your gut doesn't stay swollen. Your breath doesn't go sour. Your joints don't ache the way they used to. Your skin starts to look less tired. Your brain doesn't feel like it's wading through sludge.

You don't need a plan on top of the plan. The Hay Diet already is the plan.

Because when your food is clean and your meals digest properly, you're not storing rubbish anymore, you're clearing it. Every day. Meal by meal.

That's why this diet doesn't need a separate "detox phase." The detox is built in.

You're not doing something extreme. You're just finally stepping out of the way.

What Happens After Detox

Most people don't expect how quickly things change after the first stretch. One day you wake up and realise your stomach isn't tight. You're not bloated. You're not thinking about food. You're not foggy or sore or dragging yourself out of bed. Something just feels easier.

The system that's been overloaded for years finally gets a chance to breathe, and when it does, your body responds. The pressure starts to lift. You stop reacting to everything you eat. Your energy holds steady throughout the day. Your sleep starts to feel deeper. You stop crashing in the afternoons. You feel lighter, not just in weight, but in your head, in your chest, in how you carry yourself through the day.

You're not surviving your meals anymore. You're actually benefiting from them.

And it's not because you've perfected anything. It's just because your body finally got the room it needed to reset. You stopped mixing things that never belonged together in the first place. You stopped sending it into chaos three times a day. You let it do what it's meant to do.

You don't feel it all at once. There's no moment where everything clicks and the sun shines differently. It's more like one day, you realise you're not constantly checking how your stomach feels. You're not adjusting your waistband. You're not snapping at people for no reason halfway through the afternoon.

You eat, and then you move on. Your body handles it. No heaviness. No pressure. No crash. You get through the day without that background discomfort you'd gotten used to, the tightness, the swelling, the dragging weight you couldn't name.

Your mind stays clearer. Your skin starts to change. You notice you're more patient. You sleep better and actually wake up rested. And you didn't have to do anything extreme to get there. You just stopped forcing your body to work against itself.

That's what happens when the detox phase passes.

So if you're past day ten, and you're starting to notice these changes, lean in. This is where the momentum builds. You've done the hard bit. Now the benefits start showing up without effort. Let them carry you into the next chapter.

Chapter 7:
Transitioning into the Hay Diet

Let's drop the pressure right now, this isn't something you have to master in a day. No one's asking you to throw out everything in your kitchen and flip your life upside down before breakfast. The Hay Diet isn't a crash diet. It doesn't force a perfect routine overnight. It's a gradual shift in how you eat, and how you think about food.

Some people go all in from day one. Others take a slower path, adjusting one meal at a time. Both ways work. What matters is that you start. And then you keep going, even if it's a bit messy in the beginning.

I've seen it over and over again: people get excited, make all the changes in one go, and then crash after a week because they didn't give their body, or their mind, time to adjust. This isn't about willpower. It's about rhythm. Let your body learn its new rhythm. Give it a chance to get used to the meals, the new combinations, the lighter feeling. That takes a bit of patience.

If you've eaten a certain way your whole life, of course this will feel different. That doesn't mean it's hard. It just means it's new. And anything new feels unfamiliar until it starts to work.

Even I didn't get it perfect right away.

When I first started this diet, I didn't make some grand decision. I didn't go into the kitchen and throw everything out. I didn't tell anyone I was doing anything new. I just got tired of feeling awful and decided I couldn't keep eating the way I was.

So I made one change.

I stopped eating toast and eggs together. That was it. Same food, just not together. And it felt strange at first, because I'd done it for years. It was automatic. But I told myself, just try it this once. And I did. And after breakfast, I didn't feel bloated. I didn't feel that tight, slow heaviness I used to get by 10 a.m. I wasn't waiting for the crash or the bathroom or the next thing to go wrong. My stomach was just... fine.

That's when I realised, I didn't have to overhaul my whole life. I just had to stop making it harder for my body to cope.

So I kept going.

That's how it starts. Not with some perfectly stocked kitchen or a colour-coded plan. Just a small decision to stop doing what hasn't been working.

And if you need permission to go slow, here it is. You don't have to get it right every time. You don't have to cut everything out overnight. You just need to start choosing meals that give your system a break, and once your body starts feeling the difference, you'll want to keep going.

That's the only motivation you'll need. Relief.

This diet rewards consistency, not perfection.

So take a breath. Don't race it. Start where you are. Make one good meal. Then another. The rest will come

How to Transition

So if this doesn't need to happen overnight, then how do you actually begin?

Honestly? You begin by removing pressure. That all-or-nothing mind-set is what ruins most diets before they even start. You don't need to throw out every food you love or wake up tomorrow morning with a brand-new lifestyle. You just need to start nudging your meals in the right direction.

For me, that started with going vegetarian. Not for life. I went vegetarian for the first three months, not because I wanted to join a movement, but because it was just easier. No meat, no dairy stress, no confusion about whether I was getting the food groups wrong. Just whole grains, vegetables, lentils, fruit (at the right times), and healthy oils. That's it.

And let me be honest with you, I didn't do it because I wanted to. I did it because it made the transition easier. When you take meat out of the picture, you remove half the food combining mistakes most people make without even thinking. You can't mess up steak and potatoes if you're not eating either one. It gave my gut a breather, and it gave me time to learn the rhythm of the diet without constantly second-guessing myself.

This is how I'd suggest anyone do it:

I suggest you go on a vegetarian Hay Diet to begin with, say for the first three months. Then move onto a pescatarian diet. Then introduce chicken. Then introduce other good cuts of meat if you feel you must.

That's the exact order I followed. And I wasn't in a rush. When I added fish after a few months, it wasn't some big reward or upgrade, it was just a gentle step forward. My body was already handling the basics well, so I could start expanding without throwing things off.

After fish, I added chicken. Then, eventually, lean red meats. But by then, I already knew how my body responded to each kind of meal. I'd learned what left me feeling calm, light, and clear, and what didn't. So instead of guessing, I could actually feel what worked.

This transition doesn't require discipline. It requires patience. That's a different kind of strength. You're teaching your body a new language. And like anything new, it takes a little quiet practice before it becomes second nature.

The real change, I found, wasn't just in what I ate, it was in how I thought about food altogether. I wasn't eating reactively anymore. I wasn't reaching for whatever was in the cupboard and hoping it wouldn't upset my gut. I was choosing meals that felt aligned, that made sense, and that didn't fight each other the moment they hit my stomach.

So if you're unsure where to start, go plant-based for now. Give it a few weeks. Let it be plain and predictable. You don't need five-star recipes or Instagram-worthy plates. Just proper combinations, basic ingredients, and enough consistency for your body to catch up to what you're doing.

Then take it from there. Step by step.

Cleaning Out the Kitchen

Once you've got the mind-set right and you're easing into meals that actually make sense, it's time to look at your kitchen, because what's around you will either help or trip you up.

The truth is, most cupboards are loaded with things we don't even think twice about: sauces with hidden sugars, white bread that looks brown because it's been dyed, jars of pasta sauce with half a paragraph of ingredients you can't pronounce. It's not that any one of these things is evil, it's that together, they make it harder to stay on track. You can't follow a clean, food-combining way of eating when your shelves are working against you.

Start simple. Choose one cupboard, just one. Clear it out completely. Anything made with white flour, refined sugar, or long ingredient lists, throw it out. That includes white bread, white rice, regular pasta, snack bars pretending to be "healthy," processed cereals, and those sauces that try to sound gourmet but are packed with wheat and glucose syrup.

Now fill that cupboard with what you can eat. Stock it with:

- Wholemeal bread (real wholemeal, not coloured white bread),
- Brown rice,
- Whole grain pasta,
- Rolled oats,
- Tinned beans and lentils (no sugar added),
- Olive oil, apple cider vinegar, and lemon,
- Herbal teas,
- A few spices and dried herbs,

And vegetables that can sit on the shelf or counter, like onions, garlic, sweet potatoes.

Then move to the fridge. Keep plain yogurt, leafy greens, eggs, tofu, avocados, and clean proteins. You don't need much. Just a few basics that pair well with vegetables or stand on their own.

And remember, this isn't a one-day purge. You don't have to chuck everything at once if that stresses you out. You can phase it. Finish off what doesn't fit the plan if it makes sense, but stop replacing it. From now on, restock with intention.

There's a section I always repeat to people starting out. Before you begin, there are some things that you need to do/decide:

A) How many members of your family are going to get involved

B) You will have to get a kitchen cupboard dedicated for the Hay Diet

C) You must get rid of any sugar or salt from your cupboard

D) You should only put in your cupboard NATURAL foods"

That's it. That's the rule. It's not about having a perfect kitchen; it's about building one that doesn't fight the way you're trying to eat.

And trust me, when your shelves only contain things that work, your meals get easier. You're not wrestling with temptation or confusion every time you open the fridge. You're not wondering if this dressing or that "healthy" wrap will ruin your digestion for the next six hours.

You're just making food, eating it, and moving on with your day. That's the goal.

Keep It Simple

Once the cupboard's set up and the worst of the junk is out of the way, don't feel like you have to reinvent every meal. You don't need a brand-new meal plan for every day of the week. You just need one good meal to start with. That's it.

Pick the easiest meal of your day and clean that one up first.

For a lot of people, that's breakfast. So let's say you're used to having eggs on toast, classic combo, but a food-combining nightmare. Now you've got a choice: keep the eggs and drop the toast, or keep the toast and swap the eggs for avocado, tomato, or fruit (if you time it right).

That one swap, that one plate, can change your digestion. You'll notice your stomach feels calmer. No heaviness. No cramping two hours later. It's not a magic trick. It's just that your body doesn't have to fight to process what you gave it.

And once you've done that for a few days, move to lunch. Then dinner. Bit by bit, the puzzle pieces start fitting into place.

Don't overthink it. You're not trying to win some healthy eating award. You're just creating meals your body can actually handle. Meals that don't cancel each other out before you even finish chewing.

And yes, in the beginning, it might feel a bit repetitive. That's fine. You're not doing this to impress anyone, you're doing it to feel better. You're doing it to fix what years of mixed-up meals have broken.

I remember when I first started, I ate brown rice and steamed veg for lunch five days in a row. No sauce. Just olive oil and a pinch of salt. That meal gave me zero issues. So I kept repeating it while I figured out what else worked. It gave me a baseline. Something reliable.

You don't have to get creative right away. Just get consistent. That's what builds momentum.

Fruit Rules and Desserts

One thing that surprises people when they first try the Hay Diet is how strict it is when it comes to fruit. Not because fruit is bad, far from it, but because timing matters more than we've been told.

We've been taught to throw fruit into everything. Smoothies with milk. Fruit salad on top of yogurt. Bananas after dinner. Even diet plans will tell you fruit is the perfect dessert. But in this system, that kind of mixing causes more harm than good.

Fruit digests fast. It's light, full of water, and your body processes it quickly, *if* you eat it on an empty stomach. But once you pile it on top of a full meal, especially one with protein or starch, it doesn't go anywhere. It gets stuck. While your body's busy breaking down heavier foods, the fruit is just sitting there, fermenting. That's where the gas, bloating, and weird post-meal discomfort come from.

So, this is what I learned early on: Fruit needs space.

If you're going to eat it, do it the right way:

- Leave at least two hours after a meal before having fruit.

- Or, if you want fruit before eating, have it 30 to 60 minutes before your next meal.

This is not some picky rule to make life harder, it just gives your body the chance to digest things in the right order. You are simply letting the fastest runner leave the track first, before the slow crowd clogs it up.

When I started eating fruit on its own, away from meals, I noticed the difference immediately. No cramping. No heaviness. Just clean energy. And it didn't sit in my stomach like a rock, which is how it used to feel when I'd throw a banana on top of breakfast.

And while we're on the topic of fruit, let me clear something else up that most people get wrong.

One of the simplest pieces of advice you'll hear in nutrition is the "Five a Day" rule—the government's campaign to get people eating five portions of fruit and veg every day. But what most people don't realise is that it's five full portions; not five bites of different things. A proper portion means a handful of the same fruit or veg. So no, three strawberries, four raspberries, and half a kiwi fruit do not make three portions. That still counts as one.

When you follow the Hay Diet properly, especially with lots of neutral vegetables alongside your protein or carb meals, it becomes surprisingly easy to hit that five-a-day target without even thinking about it. You'll be eating spinach with eggs, salad with fish, and steamed veg with rice. These are all real, natural foods that actually works with your digestion, not against it. And your body will thank you for it.

Before we move forward, I'd like to clear up another misconception people have about fruit juice. A glass of pure apple juice (or any 100% pure fruit juice) does count as one of your five a day. That's important to know, especially if you're someone who finds it hard to eat whole fruits regularly.

Now, some people worry about the sugar content in these juices. But this is natural sugar, which is not harmful for your body. Your body is used to processing this type of sugar. We've been eating and drinking fruit for thousands of years, long before food labels or diet fads came along. As long as the juice is pure (not from concentrate, and with no added sugars) your system can handle it with no trouble at all.

So don't overthink it. A small glass of proper fruit juice can be a useful, easy way to tick off one of your five a day (especially if you're just starting to build better habits).

Next, let's talk about desserts. This part is uncomfortable for a lot of people, but I'll be honest.

Dessert isn't necessary. Not after meals, not right away, and definitely not if you're still adjusting to the Hay Diet.

That whole idea of finishing lunch or dinner with something sweet isn't right in the first place. That's not real hunger. That's just conditioning. Most of the time, we're not even tasting dessert. We're just chasing a feeling, sweetness, comfort, closure. But from a digestive point of view, it's a disaster.

The worst thing I used to do was finish a nice meal, one that followed all the rules, and then ruin it with a biscuit or sweet. Within minutes, I'd feel bloated and uncomfortable, like I'd undone all the good I'd just done. And that's exactly what happened. I pushed my digestion into a corner and confused the whole process.

After all those experiences, this is the truth I've come to accept:

"You should NOT have desserts after your two main meals of the day. These meal add-ons are completely unnecessary and should be avoided at all costs."

I won't blame you for being sceptical. Even, I used to think that sounded harsh. But when I stopped doing it, I realised I didn't even miss it. Not after a few weeks. Once your meals are properly combined and your blood sugar isn't spiking and crashing all the time, that urge for something sweet just fades.

Now, if you really want something like fruit or a natural sweet option, save it for mid-afternoon. Eat it on its own, well after lunch has digested. Keep it simple. Something like an apple, a few pieces of melon, or even tinned fruit in natural juice (none of that syrup stuff). But only if your last meal has had time to clear your system.

I am not asking you to give things up forever. I am just asking you to give your body the right conditions to work properly. And once that becomes your new normal, you stop craving the things that used to knock everything off balance.

Look, changing the way you eat is never just about food. It stirs things up. Mentally, emotionally, even socially. There's no point pretending this is all smooth sailing. You'll question it. You'll get frustrated. You'll open the fridge and wish you could just go back to what's easy.

That's normal.

But what I want you to hear, before you slip into the "I'll start again next week" mind-set, is this: you don't need to do this perfectly. You just need to stay with it long enough for your body to catch up.

The first week might feel weird. You'll forget some of the food combining rules. You'll second-guess a meal. You might even eat something and regret it. Don't let that throw you. This isn't a strict meal plan with points and punishments. It's a pattern of eating that works better and better the more you stick with it.

Give it three or four weeks. Not three days. Three weeks of doing your best, not aiming for gold stars, just aiming for a bit of consistency. That's when things start to change.

Your digestion starts to feel smoother. Your clothes fit better, not because you're shrinking overnight, but because the bloating's going down and your body's not holding on to junk anymore. You'll notice less heaviness after meals. Fewer crashes. Maybe even a better mood, or clearer skin. These changes creep up on you in the quiet.

That's the thing I always come back to. The real results don't scream at you. They don't show up in dramatic before-and-after shots. They show up in your normal life. In the fact that your jeans zip up without a fight. That you're not walking around half-full of air all day. That your body feels a bit more...steady.

And when you notice those changes, however small, lean into them. Let them pull you forward. You don't need motivation at that point. You've got proof.

So take the pressure off. This doesn't need to be a full kitchen makeover or a personality transplant. It just needs to start. With one clean meal. One decent shop. One day where your gut says, "Yeah, this feels better."

And if you need a reminder, know that I've been doing this for 35 years. I started just like this. I'm still here, still following the same rhythm, still feeling strong.

You can do this.

Chapter 8: Grocery Shopping and Eating Out

We've been taught to buy food by habit. You walk into the shop, grab what you always grab, trust the label, and keep moving. That's what I did for years. A loaf of brown bread that looked decent, a pack of "healthy" cereal, some sauces for convenience. It felt like I was doing the right thing. But inside my body, nothing felt right. I was still bloated, still uncomfortable after meals, still waking up heavy.

It wasn't that I was eating too much, it was that the food on my plate didn't belong together. And worse, most of it was packed with ingredients I never even noticed.

The Hay Diet forces you to slow that down. Not to make your life harder, but to help you actually feel better after you eat. That starts in the shop, not in the kitchen.

You don't need specialist aisles or health food stores. You just need to shop with your gut in mind. That means picking food that's as close to its natural state as possible, and reading the back of the packet instead of trusting the front.

For example, if we talk about brown bread. Most of it isn't brown because it's wholemeal, it's brown because it's been dyed. You turn the packet over and it's got white flour, glucose syrup, vegetable oil, preservatives, and colouring. That's not food. That's packaging pretending to be food.

I started ignoring the front and looking straight at the ingredients. Fewer words. No hidden sugars. Nothing combined in ways that would mess up digestion. That became my rule.

Shopping changed after that. I wasn't loading up a trolley with things that fought each other on the plate. I was choosing meals before I even got to the till, simple combinations I could cook without worry, because I already knew they'd sit well.

This diet doesn't push you to buy anything weird. It just asks you to think clearly before you buy what looks familiar.

The Shopping Mind-set

When I started following the Hay Diet properly, I realised that the way I was shopping had to change, not in a dramatic way, but in a more focused, deliberate one. I couldn't just walk through the aisles on autopilot anymore. I had to start noticing what I was actually bringing home.

Here's what that shift looked like for me.

I stopped buying things with long ingredient lists. If I picked something up and it had ten lines of additives, starches, sweeteners, or anything I couldn't pronounce, I put it back. That one habit made the biggest difference. Most of the stuff that sits badly in your gut comes from those packaged foods that try to cram everything into one bite, flour, sugar, oil, gums, flavourings, all in the same product. That's the kind of food that causes digestive confusion.

Instead, I kept it basic. Whole foods. Unprocessed. No extra junk mixed in. Things that didn't need fancy labels to prove they were good. Vegetables. Brown rice. Plain yogurt. Eggs. Real butter. Oats. Olive oil. That was the backbone of every shop.

And I started checking labels on things I'd trusted for years. Sauces were the worst offenders. Even the ones that claimed to be "natural" were loaded with sugar, flour, and modified starch. I used to think I was doing the right thing using a tomato-based sauce on rice or veg, until I realised it had more sweetener than a soft drink. Now I just use herbs, lemon, vinegar, or olive oil. It's not complicated. It just takes a bit more awareness.

One more thing: always go for brown over white. Brown rice. Wholemeal bread. Wholegrain pasta. But don't fall for the fake stuff, read the label. Real wholemeal flour should be listed first. Not wheat flour with colouring.

Brown bread is white bread with colouring added as we discussed above. All these wholemeal products will help your diet get back to normal, and get your guts working.

You might not believe it but It's true. Once I cut out the fake browns, my digestion actually started working properly.

Shopping like this isn't restrictive, it's just intentional. You don't need to buy a hundred different items. You just need to buy ones that won't wreck your stomach when they land on the same plate.

Staples to Keep on Hand

Once you've cleared your kitchen of the processed junk, shopping becomes much simpler. You're not chasing new products; you're stocking up on a handful of real ingredients that actually support your digestion.

Let's break it down the same way you'll build your meals: by category. Protein, carbohydrate, neutral. That's the structure. Keep it simple. Buy only what you know you'll eat, no experimenting with obscure items that sit untouched in the back of the fridge.

Protein Foods

These are the centre of your protein-based meals. Don't mix them with starches. Pair them with vegetables and healthy fats.

- Chicken (plain, skinless, no coating or marinade)
- Eggs (boiled, poached, or scrambled without milk)

- Fish (fresh or tinned in brine or olive oil)

- Tofu (plain, not sweetened or processed into fake meats)

- Natural yogurt (plain, unsweetened, no fruit added)

- Nuts and seeds (in moderation, don't go overboard)

Stick to one of these per meal. You're not combining chicken and eggs in the same plate. Keep it clean.

Carbohydrate Foods

These form the base of carb meals. No proteins here, just starch with veg and oil if needed.

- Brown rice

- Oats (plain rolled oats, not instant)

- Potatoes (boiled, baked, not fried or mashed with butter)

- Wholemeal bread (check for real wholemeal flour, not coloured white bread)

- Wholegrain pasta

- Millet, quinoa, and lentils (used in moderation and correctly combined)

You don't need massive variety here. Just one or two options that digest well for you and fit the chart.

Neutral Foods

This is the glue that ties the whole diet together. These are the only foods you can eat with either proteins *or* carbs. They help make meals taste better, feel fuller, and move easier through your system.

- Leafy greens (lettuce, spinach, rocket, kale)

- Cucumbers, courgettes, tomatoes

- Broccoli, cauliflower, cabbage

- Avocados

- Herbs and spices (dried or fresh)

- Olive oil, lemon, vinegar (natural ones, not creamy dressings)

- Garlic, ginger, onions (in small amounts)

- Non-dairy milks (unsweetened almond or oat, used sparingly)

If you've got these on hand, you can build meals easily without overthinking it. Most of the time, my plate is one main item, rice, eggs, chicken, plus two or three of these. That's it. And it works.

By following this structure, you're not trying to fill every meal with five kinds of protein or fancy sauces. Just real food that your gut can process without a fight.

Label Reading Tips

If you're serious about making this diet work, you'll need to get used to flipping products over. Not to count calories, none of that. You're flipping it over to read the ingredients. Because the front of the packet lies. That's where the marketing lives. The truth is always on the back.

That is what I look for now, and what I always missed before I started this way of eating.

Start with the length of the ingredient list. If it reads like a paragraph, put it back. Real food doesn't need to explain itself. Brown rice should say "brown rice." Nothing else. The same goes for oats, natural yogurt, tinned tomatoes. You don't need extras. You need clarity.

Next, scan for the usual suspects:

- Sugar

- Glucose syrup

- Modified starch

- Vegetable oils

- Maltodextrin

- "Flavourings" (especially when they don't tell you what kind)

- Enriched wheat flour or anything that starts with "white" or "refined"

Even so-called health foods, granola bars, salad dressings, wraps, tinned soups, are packed with this stuff. They look harmless. They're marketed as clean or organic. But once you see how much garbage is hiding inside, you realise how much better off you are cooking your own food.

And just like I said before, don't trust the word "brown" unless you see wholemeal flour listed first on the label. If it starts with wheat flour or includes caramel colour, that bread's been dyed to look healthy. That's not a whole food. That's a trick.

And when it comes to sauces, dips, soups, anything ready-made, assume it's a mess unless proven otherwise. Sugar and flour hide in places you wouldn't expect. Tomato sauce. Mustard. Stock cubes. Even some jars of olives are soaked in preservatives that disrupt digestion.

If you're not sure about something, leave it. You're better off with olive oil and lemon than some sauce pretending to be healthy.

The goal isn't to become obsessed. It's just to stay aware. A few minutes reading labels at the start saves you hours of discomfort later.

First Steps for Stocking Your Kitchen

You don't need a perfect pantry to get started. You just need one part of your kitchen that's not working against you. That's what I did, I cleared one shelf. Not the whole kitchen. Just one.

I took everything off it. All the packets of flavoured rice, instant noodles, sauces with ingredients I couldn't pronounce, biscuits I bought out of habit. Gone. I didn't even throw it all away at once. I just made a decision: nothing from that shelf goes back into my meals unless it fits the Hay Diet.

Then I restocked. Properly.

I bought brown rice. Real oats. Olive oil. A few tinned lentils. Lemons. Cucumber. Eggs. Some plain yogurt. A couple of avocados. Tomatoes. And that was enough to build a few solid meals without thinking too hard.

Start there. One shelf. A few staples. That's more than enough to give yourself options and get through the day without falling back into bad combinations.

You can build around that slowly, add a few herbs, get into the habit of boiling extra rice or prepping vegetables ahead of time. But there's no rush. The goal is to make your kitchen feel manageable, not overwhelming.

When I opened that shelf, I didn't have to think. I already knew that anything I picked from it would work. It made everything easier, less decision-making, fewer slip-ups, no "I'll just make this work" moments that used to leave me bloated and tired

That little shelf changed how I ate, how I cooked, and how I felt.

So don't wait until your kitchen is perfect. Just give yourself one reliable space. You'll be surprised how far that carries you.

Eating Out Without Stress

One of the hardest parts of changing how you eat isn't at home. It's out there, when you're not the one cooking. Someone invites you out. You're at a café with friends. You're at a wedding, or a work lunch, or a family gathering where someone's made a "nice meal" and now you've got a plate in front of you that doesn't fit the plan.

I've been there more times than I can count. And here's what I'll say: it doesn't need to be a crisis.

You don't have to explain the whole Hay Diet. You don't need to ask for a new meal or draw attention to yourself. You just need to manage your plate quietly and move on.

"When I go out for a meal, if there is anything on the plate I can't eat with the rest of the meal, such as potatoes, I just make up an excuse that I was too full to eat them."

That's it. No debate. No scene. Just a simple, polite line like:

- "I'm full, I'll leave that bit."

- "That hasn't been sitting well with me lately."

- "I've been eating lighter, that's all."

Nobody cares as much as you think they do. Most of the time, people don't even notice.

Here's the basic rule when you're eating out: **pick your base.** Either you go for a protein-based meal, or a carb-based one, not both. That's your anchor. Then build around it with neutral foods like vegetables, salad, or olive oil.

If you're having grilled chicken, skip the potatoes and ask for extra veg. If you're going for pasta, skip the cheese or meat and ask for olive oil and herbs instead of creamy sauce. Most restaurants won't blink at that kind of request. You're not being fussy. You're just choosing what works for your body.

And if something shows up on the plate that doesn't belong, just leave it. You don't owe anyone an explanation. You're looking after your health, not performing for the table.

This way of eating was never meant to isolate you. It's not a social punishment. You can still enjoy meals out, still sit at a table with others, still have a good time. You just do it with a bit of awareness and a few polite boundaries. No obsession. No stress.

What matters isn't perfection, it's the pattern. You can't control every plate, but you can control your choices on it.

You're going to mess up. Let's just say that now.

You'll eat the wrong combination. You'll forget what's neutral. You'll be halfway through a meal and realise there's flour in the sauce or sugar in the dressing. And you'll wonder, *does this ruin everything?*

It doesn't.

This isn't a test. There's no grade at the end. The Hay Diet isn't something you pass or fail, it's something you get better at by doing. What matters isn't whether you got every bite right. What matters is whether you keep showing up for the next one.

The people who get results aren't the ones who followed the rules perfectly. They're the ones who kept going even after they slipped. They didn't let one bad meal become an excuse to quit. They just moved on and did the next meal properly.

That's what makes it work in real life.

You're not aiming for clean eating with no mistakes forever. You're aiming for consistency. That's where the change happens. Not in a single perfect day, but in a dozen ordinary ones done mostly right.

And here's the truth, once you start feeling better, it gets easier to stick with it. The bloating fades. Your energy comes back. You start noticing which foods make you feel lighter, clearer, more awake. And then it's not about willpower anymore. It's just how you eat now.

Slip-ups don't break the system. Giving up does.

So take the pressure off. Focus on what you're doing right. Keep your meals clean when you can. And when you can't, don't panic, just come back to what you know.

That's how you make it last.

Chapter 9: Weekly Meal Planning

Meal planning has a bad reputation. Most people think it means eating the same thing every day or measuring out food like you're prepping for a science experiment. But that's not what we're doing here. The whole point of the Hay Diet is to take pressure off your digestion, not to pile it onto your schedule.

Planning your meals ahead of time is just a way to make this diet easier to follow. That's it. It's not restrictive. It's not rigid. It's just preparation. You're building a rhythm so that when you're tired, distracted, or short on time, you've still got something that works. Something that won't undo your progress.

And it starts with something simple: three meals a day. No grazing. No snacking every hour. Just three balanced meals, spaced out, properly combined.

"Your meals should be three meals a day; Breakfast, lunch and dinner."

That one line changed the way I ate. It gave my gut time to rest between meals instead of being stuck in constant processing mode.

The structure looks like this:

- Breakfast is either carbohydrate-based or fruit-based.

- Lunch is your protein-focused meal.

- Dinner is light and flexible, usually built around vegetables, with either a little protein or carbs, depending on the day.

Once you get used to that flow, you'll find it gives you energy, not drains it. You won't be hungry all the time because your meals actually digest properly and leave you satisfied.

Now that you know the daily rhythm, three meals, properly spaced, with the right combinations, it's time to make it practical.

Before this, I didn't really plan meals at all. I ate what I felt like, when I felt like it. Breakfast was whatever I could grab. Lunch was often something quick or random. Dinner was a mix of everything I thought I needed to feel full. Looking back, most of my meals were just a pile of good and bad combinations thrown together, and I had no idea why I kept feeling heavy, bloated, or foggy after eating.

So when I started following the Hay Diet properly, I realised that planning wasn't about restriction, it was about making things easier. I wasn't trying to follow a strict schedule or make every day look the same. I just needed to stop guessing. I needed a basic rhythm that would work even on days when I didn't feel like thinking.

That's when I started sticking to the three-meal flow.

- Breakfast: Carb-based or fruit-based. Not both. Not mixed. Just something light and digestible to start the day without upsetting my stomach.
- Lunch: Always protein-focused. It became my main meal. Clean proteins paired with vegetables or neutral foods.
- Dinner: Lighter, easier, and flexible, usually based around vegetables, with a little protein or a small amount of carbs, depending on how the day went.

This setup gave my body time to digest, rest, and reset between meals. No snacking, no food overlaps, no confusion. Just clear, balanced structure.

And to make it even easier, I started rotating between carb days and protein days. This is what that looks like in real life.

Sample Day: Carbohydrate-Focused

- Breakfast: Wholemeal toast with mashed avocado and sliced tomato. It's filling, gentle, and easy to prepare. No heavy proteins. Just clean carbs paired with neutrals that digest smoothly.

- Lunch: Brown rice with steamed broccoli and a drizzle of olive oil. Nothing fancy. Just three ingredients that sit well together. It gives energy without the crash or the fog.

- Dinner: Homemade vegetable soup with oat crackers and cucumber slices. Light enough for the evening. Easy on digestion. If you've had a busy day, this kind of meal won't weigh you down.

- Fruit snack: A banana or an apple, but only in the late afternoon, between meals. If I'd just eaten lunch or dinner, I'd hold off for a couple of hours. Let the stomach clear before introducing fruit.

This kind of day is ideal when I want something grounding but not too heavy. It keeps me regular, keeps my head clear, and gives me steady energy.

Sample Day: Protein-Focused

- Breakfast: Two boiled eggs with lightly sautéed spinach It's clean, satisfying, and holds you through the morning without spiking your blood sugar.

- Lunch: Grilled chicken with a fresh salad, lettuce, cucumber, a bit of lemon juice and olive oil I keep it basic. No cheese, no bread on the side. Just protein and neutral veg. That's what works.

- Dinner: Zucchini noodles with olive oil, herbs, and maybe a bit of garlic. No pasta. No bread. Just something that feels like a proper meal but doesn't interfere with sleep or digestion.

- Fruit snack: A small bowl of tinned peaches in natural juice, not syrup. I'll have this a couple hour after lunch if I feel like eating something sweet. Not with the meal though and definitely not right after.

This protein focused day works well when I want to feel stronger or more mentally alert. The meals are simple, but they leave no digestive confusion behind. That's the part I never used to pay attention to, the feeling *after* the meal.

You don't need a dozen new recipes every week. You don't need to cook differently every night. What you need are meals that feel good, meals that your body can actually process without punishment.

These examples aren't the limit. They're just a starting point. Once you get the rhythm, you'll be able to swap ingredients in and out without second-guessing. That's the freedom. You build your own version of this diet based on meals that actually work for you.

And that all starts with keeping it simple.

If there's one rule that trips people up without them realising it, it's fruit. Not because fruit is bad. Not because it's too sugary. But because it's almost always eaten at the wrong time.

I used to eat fruit whenever I felt like it, after meals, as a quick snack, even mixed into things like yogurt or cereal. It felt like a healthy choice. It never crossed my mind that timing mattered.

But once I started paying attention, I noticed the pattern. I'd have a big lunch, feel fine, then eat a piece of fruit half an hour later and suddenly feel bloated, gassy or weirdly full. At first I blamed the meal. It took me a while to realise, it was the fruit.

Here's the thing: fruit digests fast. Much faster than anything else on your plate. So if you eat it after a heavier meal, especially one with protein or starch, it gets stuck. Your stomach's already busy dealing with slower-digesting food, and the fruit just sits there on top of it all, fermenting. That's where the discomfort starts.

So I made one change:
I only ate fruit on its own.
At least two hours after a meal, or 30 to 60 minutes before the next one like I discussed in chapter 7.

It was a small adjustment, but it made a huge difference. Fruit stopped giving me issues. It felt light again. Energising. Clean. And because I wasn't layering it on top of other food, it didn't throw off my digestion.

Let's talk about desserts next.

Most people expect some kind of sweet finish after lunch or dinner. Not because they're hungry, but because they're used to it. It's habit. But if you're serious about making this diet work, this is one habit you've got to break.

Desserts don't belong at the end of a meal. Especially not one that already includes protein or carbs. All they do is overload your gut when it's already full. And when that happens, everything slows down. Digestion backs up. Bloating, tiredness, and heaviness creep in. You feel like you undid the whole meal, and in a way, you did.

"You should NOT have desserts after your two main meals of the day. These meal add-ons are completely unnecessary and should be avoided at all costs."

And that's the truth. Not because desserts are evil. But because your body doesn't need more food right after it's started working on what you just gave it.

If you want something sweet, have fruit. But have it later. Between meals. On its own. That's how it gives you energy without messing up everything else.

Once I got used to eating this way, I didn't miss desserts. My cravings faded. My digestion felt smoother. And food started giving me energy instead of taking it.

That's the whole point.

Practical Planning Tips

Meal planning isn't about turning your life into a routine. It's about giving yourself fewer decisions to make when you're tired, busy, or just not in the mood to think. The more of that guesswork you can take out of the day, the easier this diet becomes.

The first thing I did was prep a few basics that I could fall back on. Nothing complicated, just a few ingredients I always had ready. Boiled eggs. Cooked brown rice. A container of chopped veg. A few pieces of fruit. That was enough to build something decent without having to start from scratch every time.

You don't need a meal plan written out hour by hour. You just need a few meals you trust. Ones you know won't leave you bloated or uncomfortable. I had two or three for breakfast, a couple for lunch, and a few easy dinners I could throw together in ten minutes. That was it.

I also kept one shelf in the fridge and one in the cupboard stocked with Hay-friendly ingredients. If something ran out, I replaced it on my next shop. If I had a long day ahead, I'd make my lunch the night before, grilled chicken and cucumber, or a bowl of brown rice with lemon and broccoli. I wasn't trying to be perfect. I was just making the next day easier.

And when I had energy, I'd cook in bigger batches. A pot of soup that would last a few dinners. A tray of roasted vegetables I could use with lunch for the next few days. Those kinds of small steps save you on the days when nothing else goes to plan.

Some people like to make a chart or a printed list. If that helps, do it. But it's not essential. What matters is finding your rhythm. Knowing what works for your body, and being ready for the days when motivation isn't going to carry you.

This way of eating doesn't need to be rigid. But it does need consistency. That's what keeps your digestion steady. That's what helps you feel in control when everything else is moving around you.

Don't overcomplicate it. Just plan enough to stay clear, and let that carry you forward.

People get stuck when they try to make every meal flawless. They aim for the perfect plate, the perfect routine, the perfect day, and when one thing goes off track, they think they've ruined it. So they give up. Or start again next Monday. Or let one slip turn into three days of chaos.

That's not how this works.

The Hay Diet doesn't expect perfection. It asks for rhythm. It asks you to show up again and again, not because you're being strict, but because your body *needs that kind of steadiness* to work properly.

You're trying to rebuild your digestion. And that's not something that happens in one great week. It happens when you stay consistent. When your gut stops being surprised by your food. When your meals don't change tone or structure every other day.

You might mess up a food combination here and there. You might forget to time fruit properly. That's okay. What matters is that you go back to the plan at the next meal, not next week, not when it's convenient. Just the next meal.

There were times I didn't have the right ingredients. Times I ate out and guessed wrong. But I didn't throw the whole thing out because of it. I kept the rhythm going. And over time, it got easier. The meals became second nature. The planning wasn't effort anymore; it was just how I ate.

That's the place you're aiming for. Not perfection. Just enough consistency that your body learns to trust what's coming next.

You'll still have days when things don't go to plan. That's life. But the meals you've already cleaned up, the good ones you repeat, the habits that are starting to stick, they're doing more for you than you realise.

Chapter 10: Hay Diet Recipes

You don't need complicated meals to feel better. You need combinations that don't wreck your digestion. That's what these recipes are for.

This isn't a recipe book full of exotic ingredients or fancy prep. These are the meals that actually work, simple, repeatable, properly combined. Meals you can cook without second-guessing. Meals that won't leave you bloated or tired an hour later.

I'm not giving you 50 variations of the same thing. I'm giving you a handful of meals that you can rely on. Things I've eaten for years. No gimmicks, no weird flour substitutes, no sweeteners pretending to be natural. Just normal food that keeps your gut working and your energy steady.

Some are protein-based. Some are carb-based. None of them mix the wrong things together. All of them are built around the food combining chart you've already learned.

If you've made it this far, you don't need to be told what to do, you just need a few examples to make it easier. That's what this chapter will give you. Let's start with the protein based recipes.

Protein-Based Recipes

Before I start sharing the recipes, I'd like to remind you about the fruit rule again. Please do not eat fruit directly after this meal. If you want fruit, have it on its own, either 30 minutes before or at least 2 hours later. Combining fruit with protein can interfere with digestion and slow things down.

Spinach & Mushroom Omelette with Fresh Herbs

What you need:

- 2 large eggs
- 1 cup fresh spinach, roughly chopped
- ½ cup mushrooms, thinly sliced (any kind, I usually go with button or chestnut)
- 1 tablespoon olive oil or a knob of butter
- Fresh parsley or chives, chopped (optional but makes it nicer)
- Salt and black pepper to taste

How to make it:

1. Crack the eggs into a bowl and beat them well with a pinch of salt and black pepper. Set aside.

2. Heat the olive oil or butter in a non-stick pan over medium heat.

3. Toss in the mushrooms first. Let them cook for about 4–5 minutes until they've softened and started to brown. Don't rush this part, mushrooms need time to release their moisture.

4. Add the spinach. Stir gently until it wilts down. This should take about a minute or two.

5. Once the veggies are cooked, spread them out evenly in the pan and pour the eggs on top.

6. Let it cook undisturbed for a minute or two. Tilt the pan occasionally to let uncooked egg slide underneath.

7. Once the eggs are nearly set, sprinkle your herbs over the top. Fold one side over to make a half-moon shape.

8. Cook for another 30 seconds, then slide it onto a plate.

Serve with:

A few slices of fresh tomato, cucumber, or a handful of salad leaves dressed with lemon juice and a splash of olive oil. No toast or bread, that would break the Hay Diet rules.

Why this works for the Hay Diet:

Eggs are protein.
Spinach, mushrooms, herbs are neutral foods.
Olive oil is neutral fat.
Everything on the plate supports digestion, keeps the meal light, and avoids the protein-carb clash.

Optional Tips:

- You can double the quantity for two people.

- If prepping ahead, cook the mushrooms and spinach, store them in a container, and add to eggs when needed.

- Don't pair this with fruit, wait 2 hours before or after to eat any.

Storage Tip:

This is best eaten fresh, but if needed, you can store it in the fridge for up to 24 hours and gently reheat on the pan.

Grilled Lemon Herb Salmon with Steamed Greens

What you need:

- 1 salmon fillet (about 6 oz or 170g)

- Juice of half a lemon
- 1 tablespoon olive oil
- 1 garlic clove, minced
- Fresh herbs (such as dill, parsley, or thyme), chopped
- Salt and black pepper to taste
- A handful of green beans or asparagus
- A wedge of lemon, for serving

How to make it:

1. In a small bowl, mix the lemon juice, olive oil, minced garlic, and chopped herbs to create a marinade.

2. Place the salmon fillet in a shallow dish and pour the marinade over it. Let it sit for at least 15 minutes to absorb the flavors.

3. While the salmon is marinating, steam the green beans or asparagus until tender but still crisp, about 4-5 minutes. Set aside.

4. Preheat your grill or grill pan over medium heat. Once hot, place the salmon skin-side down and cook for about 4-5 minutes per side, depending on thickness, until the fish is opaque and flakes easily with a fork.

5. Serve the grilled salmon alongside the steamed greens, with a wedge of lemon on the side for an extra burst of freshness.

Serving Suggestion:

This dish pairs wonderfully with a simple green salad dressed in olive oil and lemon juice. Remember, no starchy sides like potatoes or rice to keep in line with the Hay Diet principles.

Why this works for the Hay Diet:

Salmon is a protein-rich food, and when combined with neutral vegetables like green beans or asparagus, it aligns perfectly with the Hay Diet's food combining rules. Avoiding starchy accompaniments ensures better digestion and nutrient absorption.

Optional Tips:

- For added flavor, sprinkle some capers over the salmon before serving.

- If you prefer baking, wrap the marinated salmon in foil and bake at 375°F (190°C) for about 15-20 minutes.

Lemon-Herb Grilled Chicken with Steamed Broccoli

What you need:

- 1 boneless, skinless chicken breast (about 6 oz or 170g)

- Juice of 1 lemon

- 2 tablespoons olive oil

- 2 garlic cloves, minced

- 1 teaspoon dried oregano (or fresh, if available)

- Salt and black pepper to taste

- 1 cup broccoli florets

How to make it:

1. In a bowl, whisk together the lemon juice, olive oil, minced garlic, oregano, salt, and pepper to create a marinade.

2. Place the chicken breast in a shallow dish and pour the marinade over it. Cover and refrigerate for at least 30 minutes, allowing the flavours to infuse.

3. While the chicken is marinating, steam the broccoli florets until tender but still crisp, about 4-5 minutes. Set aside.

4. Preheat your grill or grill pan over medium heat. Remove the chicken from the marinade and grill for about 6-7 minutes on each side, or until the internal temperature reaches 165°F (74°C) and the juices run clear.

5. Let the chicken rest for a few minutes before slicing.

Serving Suggestion:
Serve the grilled chicken alongside the steamed broccoli. For added flavor, drizzle a bit of the remaining marinade over the broccoli (ensure it's been cooked to eliminate any raw chicken contamination) or squeeze a fresh lemon wedge over the entire dish.

Why this works for the Hay Diet:
Chicken is a protein-rich food, and when paired with neutral vegetables like broccoli, it adheres to the Hay Diet's food combining rules. This combination supports optimal digestion and nutrient absorption.

Optional Tips:

- For variety, substitute broccoli with other neutral vegetables like zucchini or green beans.

- Add fresh herbs like parsley or basil for an extra burst of flavor.

Herb-Crusted Baked Cod with Steamed Zucchini

What you need:

- 1 cod fillet (about 6 oz or 170g)

- 1 tablespoon olive oil

- 1 teaspoon Dijon mustard

- 1 tablespoon fresh parsley, chopped

- 1 teaspoon fresh thyme leaves

- 1 garlic clove, minced

- Zest of half a lemon

- Salt and black pepper to taste

- 1 medium zucchini, sliced into rounds

How to make it:

1. Preheat your oven to 400°F (200°C).

2. In a small bowl, mix the olive oil, Dijon mustard, chopped parsley, thyme, minced garlic, lemon zest, salt, and pepper to create the herb mixture.

3. Place the cod fillet on a baking sheet lined with parchment paper. Spread the herb mixture evenly over the top of the fillet.

4. Bake in the preheated oven for 12-15 minutes, or until the fish flakes easily with a fork.

5. While the cod is baking, steam the zucchini slices until tender, about 4-5 minutes.

6. Serve the herb-crusted cod alongside the steamed zucchini.

Serving Suggestion:
Drizzle a bit of fresh lemon juice over the cod and zucchini for

an extra burst of flavour. A simple green salad with a light vinaigrette can also complement this meal well.

Why this works for the Hay Diet:
Cod is a lean protein, and when paired with neutral vegetables like zucchini, it adheres to the Hay Diet's food combining rules. The absence of starchy sides ensures better digestion and nutrient absorption.

Optional Tips:

- For added flavour, consider adding a pinch of chili flakes to the herb mixture.

- If fresh herbs aren't available, dried herbs can be used, but reduce the quantity by half.

Cottage Cheese & Herb-Stuffed Bell Peppers

What you need:

- 2 large bell peppers (any colour), halved and seeds removed

- 1 cup cottage cheese (preferably low-fat)

- 1 tablespoon fresh parsley, chopped

- 1 tablespoon fresh dill, chopped

- 1 garlic clove, minced

- Salt and black pepper to taste

- 1 teaspoon olive oil

- Optional: a sprinkle of paprika for garnish

How to make it:

1. Preheat your oven to 375°F (190°C).

2. In a bowl, combine the cottage cheese, chopped herbs, minced garlic, salt, and pepper. Mix well to incorporate all the flavours.

3. Lightly brush the bell pepper halves with olive oil.

4. Spoon the cottage cheese mixture into each bell pepper half, filling them generously.

5. Place the stuffed peppers in a baking dish and bake for 20-25 minutes, or until the peppers are tender and the filling is heated through.

6. Remove from the oven and, if desired, sprinkle a bit of paprika on top for added colour and flavour.

Serving Suggestion:
Serve these stuffed peppers warm, accompanied by a side of mixed greens dressed with lemon juice and olive oil.

Why this works for the Hay Diet:
Cottage cheese is a protein-rich food, and when paired with neutral vegetables like bell peppers and herbs, it adheres to the Hay Diet's food combining rules. This combination supports optimal digestion and nutrient absorption.

Optional Tips:

• For added texture, consider mixing in some finely chopped celery or cucumber into the cottage cheese filling.

• These stuffed peppers can also be enjoyed cold, making them a great option for meal prep or on-the-go lunches.

• This dish keeps well. Store in the fridge for up to 2 days and enjoy cold or at room temperature. Great for lunchboxes too.

Baked Tofu with Garlic-Ginger Glaze and Steamed Bok Choy

This Asian-inspired dish is a delightful combination of baked tofu infused with a savoury garlic-ginger glaze, paired with steamed bok choy. It's light, satisfying, and perfectly aligned with the Hay Diet's food combining principles.

What you need:

- 1 block (14 oz or 400g) firm tofu, drained and pressed
- 2 tablespoons tamari or low-sodium soy sauce
- 1 tablespoon sesame oil
- 1 tablespoon fresh ginger, grated
- 2 garlic cloves, minced
- 1 tablespoon rice vinegar
- 1 teaspoon maple syrup or honey (optional for a hint of sweetness)
- 1 tablespoon sesame seeds
- 2 heads of bok choy, halved lengthwise
- Salt and black pepper to taste

How to make it:

1. Preheat your oven to 400°F (200°C).

2. Cut the pressed tofu into 1-inch cubes and place them in a shallow dish.

3. In a small bowl, whisk together tamari, sesame oil, grated ginger, minced garlic, rice vinegar, and maple syrup or honey if using.

4. Pour the marinade over the tofu cubes, ensuring they are well-coated. Let them marinate for at least 15 minutes.

5. Place the marinated tofu cubes on a baking sheet lined with parchment paper. Bake for 25-30 minutes, turning halfway through, until golden and slightly crispy.

6. While the tofu is baking, steam the bok choy halves until tender, about 5-7 minutes.

7. Serve the baked tofu over the steamed bok choy, garnished with sesame seeds.

Serving Suggestion:

This dish pairs well with a side of cucumber salad dressed in rice vinegar and sesame oil.

Why this works for the Hay Diet:

Tofu is a protein-rich food, and when paired with neutral vegetables like bok choy, it adheres to the Hay Diet's food combining rules. This combination supports optimal digestion and nutrient absorption.

Optional Tips:

- For added flavour, sprinkle chopped green onions or cilantro over the dish before serving.

- If you prefer a spicier kick, add a dash of chili flakes to the marinade.

- This dish keeps well. Store in the fridge for up to 2 days and enjoy cold or at room temperature. Great for lunchboxes too.

Grilled Chicken Salad with Lemon-Herb Dressing

What you need:

- 1 boneless, skinless chicken breast (about 6 oz or 170g)

- 1 tablespoon olive oil

- Juice of 1 lemon

- 1 garlic clove, minced

- 1 teaspoon fresh thyme leaves

- Salt and black pepper to taste

- 4 cups mixed salad greens (e.g., romaine, arugula, spinach)

- 1/2 cucumber, sliced

- 1/2 red bell pepper, sliced

- 1/4 red onion, thinly sliced

How to make it:

1. In a small bowl, mix the olive oil, lemon juice, minced garlic, thyme, salt, and pepper to create the marinade.

2. Place the chicken breast in a shallow dish and pour half of the marinade over it. Let it marinate for at least 30 minutes. Reserve the other half of the marinade for the dressing.

3. Preheat your grill or grill pan over medium heat. Remove the chicken from the marinade and grill for about 6-7 minutes on each side, or until the internal temperature reaches 165°F (74°C).

4. Let the chicken rest for a few minutes before slicing it thinly.

5. In a large bowl, combine the salad greens, cucumber, red bell pepper, and red onion.

6. Top the salad with the sliced grilled chicken and drizzle with the reserved lemon-herb dressing.

Serving Suggestion:

Serve this salad on its own for a light meal, or pair it with a side of steamed green beans or asparagus for added variety.

Why this works for the Hay Diet:

Chicken is a protein-rich food, and when paired with neutral vegetables like salad greens, cucumber, and bell peppers, it adheres to the Hay Diet's food combining rules. This combination supports optimal digestion and nutrient absorption.

Optional Tips:

- For added flavour, sprinkle some chopped fresh parsley or basil over the salad before serving.

- If you prefer a bit of heat, add a pinch of red pepper flakes to the dressing.

- This dish keeps well. Store in the fridge for up to 3 days and enjoy cold or at room temperature. Great for lunchboxes too.

Grilled Turkey Breast with Steamed Green Beans

What you need:

- 1 turkey breast fillet (about 6 oz or 170g)

- 1 tablespoon olive oil

- Juice of half a lemon

- 1 garlic clove, minced

- 1 teaspoon fresh rosemary, chopped

- Salt and black pepper to taste

- 1 cup green beans, trimmed

How to make it:

1. In a small bowl, mix the olive oil, lemon juice, minced garlic, chopped rosemary, salt, and pepper to create a marinade.

2. Place the turkey breast in a shallow dish and pour the marinade over it. Let it marinate for at least 30 minutes.

3. Preheat your grill or grill pan over medium heat. Remove the turkey from the marinade and grill for about 6-7 minutes on each side, or until the internal temperature reaches 165°F (74°C).

4. While the turkey is grilling, steam the green beans until tender but still crisp, about 4-5 minutes.

5. Serve the grilled turkey breast alongside the steamed green beans.

Serving Suggestion:

For added flavour, drizzle a bit of the remaining marinade over the green beans before serving.

Why this works for the Hay Diet:

Turkey is a lean protein, and when paired with neutral vegetables like green beans, it adheres to the Hay Diet's food combining rules. This combination supports optimal digestion and nutrient absorption.

Optional Tips:

- For variety, substitute green beans with other neutral vegetables like zucchini or asparagus.

- Add fresh herbs like parsley or thyme for an extra burst of flavour.

- This dish keeps well. Store in the fridge for up to 3 days and enjoy cold or at room temperature. Great for lunchboxes too.

Grilled Lamb Chops with Minted Courgette Ribbons

What you need:

- 2 lamb chops (about 6 oz or 170g each)

- 1 tablespoon olive oil

- 2 garlic cloves, minced

- 1 teaspoon fresh rosemary, chopped

- Salt and black pepper to taste

- 2 medium courgettes (zucchini), sliced into ribbons using a vegetable peeler

- Juice of half a lemon

- 1 tablespoon fresh mint, chopped

How to make it:

1. In a small bowl, mix the olive oil, minced garlic, chopped rosemary, salt, and pepper to create a marinade.

2. Place the lamb chops in a shallow dish and pour the marinade over them. Let them marinate for at least 30 minutes to absorb the flavours.

3. Preheat your grill or grill pan over medium-high heat. Remove the lamb chops from the marinade and grill for

about 4-5 minutes on each side, or until they reach your desired level of doneness.

4. While the lamb is grilling, bring a pot of water to a boil. Blanch the courgette ribbons for about 1 minute, then drain and pat dry.

5. In a bowl, toss the courgette ribbons with lemon juice and chopped mint. Season with a pinch of salt and pepper.

6. Serve the grilled lamb chops alongside the minted courgette ribbons.

Serving Suggestion:

For added freshness, garnish the dish with a few extra mint leaves and a lemon wedge on the side.

Why this works for the Hay Diet:

Lamb is a protein-rich food, and when paired with neutral vegetables like courgettes, it adheres to the Hay Diet's food combining rules. This combination supports optimal digestion and nutrient absorption.

Optional Tips:

- If you prefer, you can pan-sear the lamb chops instead of grilling them.

- For a touch of sweetness, add a drizzle of honey to the courgette ribbons

Baked Haddock with Lemon-Dill Sauce and Steamed Asparagus

What you need:

- 1 haddock fillet (about 6 oz or 170g)
- 1 tablespoon olive oil
- Juice of half a lemon
- 1 teaspoon fresh dill, chopped
- 1 garlic clove, minced
- Salt and black pepper to taste
- 1 cup asparagus spears, trimmed

How to make it:

1. Preheat your oven to 375°F (190°C).
2. Place the haddock fillet on a baking sheet lined with parchment paper.
3. In a small bowl, mix the olive oil, lemon juice, chopped dill, minced garlic, salt, and pepper.
4. Drizzle the lemon-dill mixture over the haddock fillet.
5. Bake the haddock for 15-20 minutes, or until the fish flakes easily with a fork.
6. While the fish is baking, steam the asparagus spears until tender but still crisp, about 4-5 minutes.
7. Serve the baked haddock alongside the steamed asparagus.

Serving Suggestion:

For added flavor, garnish the dish with additional fresh dill and lemon wedges.

Why this works for the Hay Diet:

Haddock is a lean protein, and when paired with neutral vegetables like asparagus, it adheres to the Hay Diet's food combining rules. This combination supports optimal digestion and nutrient absorption.

Optional Tips:

- If haddock is unavailable, you can substitute it with other white fish like cod or pollock.

- For a touch of heat, add a pinch of red pepper flakes to the lemon-dill sauce.

Carbohydrate-Based Recipes

When most people think "carbs," they picture something heavy, bread, pasta, potatoes, and instantly worry it'll make them feel bloated or sluggish. But here's the truth: carbohydrates aren't the problem. Bad combinations are.

On the Hay Diet, we don't cut out carbs. We just give them space to digest properly. That means you don't pair them with protein (like cheese, meat, or eggs), but with neutral foods like vegetables, herbs, and healthy oils. Once you do that, something strange happens, your meals feel lighter, your stomach stops swelling up, and your energy lasts longer.

These next recipes are all based on that logic. Each one features a single starchy base, like brown rice, oats, potatoes, or wholemeal pasta, paired with neutral ingredients to keep your digestion flowing. They're filling but easy on the gut, and you'll actually feel good after eating them.

Let's start simple:

Brown Rice with Stir-Fried Cabbage and Carrot

What you need:

- 75g brown rice (uncooked)

- 1 tablespoon olive oil

- 1 garlic clove, finely chopped

- ½ small cabbage, thinly sliced

- 1 medium carrot, julienned or grated

- 1 teaspoon sesame seeds (optional)

- Salt and black pepper to taste

How to make it:

1. Rinse the brown rice and cook it in double the volume of water (about 150ml) for 20–25 minutes until tender. Drain any excess water.

2. While the rice is cooking, heat olive oil in a pan. Add the garlic and stir for 30 seconds.

3. Toss in the sliced cabbage and carrot. Stir-fry for about 5–7 minutes until just softened but still vibrant.

4. Season with salt, pepper, and sesame seeds if using.

5. Serve the stir-fried veg over the cooked rice.

Neutral Pairing Tip:
If you want a fresh side, a cucumber salad with lemon juice works beautifully. Just keep it neutral, no cheese, yogurt, or creamy sauces.

Fruit Reminder:
Don't follow this with fruit. Give your body a 2-hour window before adding anything sweet. Or if you're hungry later, have fruit on its own.

Storage Tip:
You can batch this ahead. Store in the fridge for up to 3 days. Best served warm, but still good cold in a packed lunch.

Why this works for the Hay Diet:
Brown rice is your starch, cabbage and carrot are neutral. No protein involved so no conflict. It's filling but leaves your digestion calm and comfortable.

Baked Sweet Potato with Olive Oil and Fresh Herbs

What you need:

- 1 medium sweet potato (around 200g)

- 1 tablespoon olive oil

- A small handful of fresh parsley or coriander, chopped

- Pinch of sea salt and black pepper

- Optional: squeeze of lemon or a pinch of paprika

How to make it:

1. Preheat your oven to 200°C (fan 180°C).

2. Scrub the sweet potato clean but leave the skin on. Prick a few holes in it with a fork.

3. Place on a baking tray and bake for 40–45 minutes, or until soft and caramelised inside.

4. Once baked, slice it open and drizzle with olive oil. Sprinkle with salt, pepper, herbs, and any optional extras you like.

Neutral Pairing Tip:
You can add a spoonful of sautéed spinach or a simple side salad of rocket, cucumber, and lemon juice, just keep it light and protein-free.

Fruit Reminder:

No fruit with this meal. Wait 2 hours if you want some later. Combining fruit with starch can slow down digestion and leave you bloated.

Storage Tip:

You can bake a few sweet potatoes at once and keep them in the fridge for up to 3 days. Reheat in the oven or enjoy cold with olive oil and herbs.

Why this works for the Hay Diet:

Sweet potato is carbohydrate. Everything else, herbs, olive oil, leafy greens, is neutral. No protein means no digestive clash, just clean energy and comfort.

Wholemeal Pasta with Garlic-Roasted Vegetables

What you need:

- 75g wholemeal pasta
- 1 tablespoon olive oil
- 1 courgette, sliced
- 1 red pepper, chopped
- 1 small red onion, sliced
- 2 garlic cloves, minced
- 1 teaspoon dried oregano
- Salt and black pepper

How to make it:

1. Preheat the oven to 200°C (fan 180°C).

2. In a roasting tray, combine the courgette, pepper, onion, and garlic. Drizzle with olive oil, sprinkle with oregano, season with salt and pepper, and toss to coat.

3. Roast for 20 to 25 minutes, stirring halfway through, until the vegetables are tender and slightly caramelised.

4. While the veg is roasting, cook the pasta according to the packet instructions. Drain and set aside.

5. Combine the roasted vegetables with the pasta and toss gently. Serve warm. Fresh basil on top is a nice touch if you have it.

Neutral pairing tip:
This works well with a side salad of rocket and cucumber dressed in lemon juice and olive oil. Keep it simple. Don't add cheese or protein, that's what throws digestion off.

Fruit timing:
Do not follow this with fruit. If you plan to have fruit, eat it at least 30 minutes before this meal or wait a full 2 hours after.

Storage:
Keeps well in the fridge for up to 2 days. Can be reheated or eaten cold as a pasta salad.

Why it works for the Hay Diet:
Pasta is carb. Vegetables and herbs is neutral. No protein involved. That means your stomach can digest it without conflict or strain.

Quinoa Salad with Cucumber, Tomato, and Mint

What you need:

- 70g quinoa

- 150ml water

- ½ cucumber, diced

- 1 medium tomato, diced

- Juice of half a lemon

- 1 tablespoon olive oil

- A small handful of fresh mint, finely chopped

- Salt and black pepper

How to make it:

1. Rinse the quinoa under cold water, then place it in a saucepan with the water.

2. Bring to a boil, then reduce the heat and simmer gently with the lid on for 12 to 15 minutes, or until the water is absorbed and the quinoa is fluffy.

3. Let it sit, covered, for another 5 minutes, then fluff with a fork and allow to cool slightly.

4. In a bowl, mix the cooled quinoa with cucumber, tomato, lemon juice, olive oil, chopped mint, salt, and pepper.

5. Stir well and let it sit for 5–10 minutes so the flavours come together. Serve at room temperature or slightly chilled.

Neutral pairing tip:
You can serve this with a side of leafy greens or steamed courgette. Don't add cheese or beans, they'll turn it into a mixing mess.

Fruit timing:
Avoid eating fruit with this or straight after. Wait at least two hours if you want fruit later, or have fruit 30 minutes before this meal.

Storage:

This keeps well in the fridge for up to 2 days. It's perfect for lunchboxes or a quick dinner you don't have to overthink.

Why it works for the Hay Diet:

Quinoa is your starch here. Everything else, vegetables, lemon juice, herbs, and olive oil, is neutral. You're keeping it simple, letting each food digest in its own lane.

Boiled Potatoes with Olive Oil and Dill

What you need:

- 200g small new potatoes (such as baby or Charlotte)
- 1 tablespoon olive oil
- 1 tablespoon fresh dill, finely chopped
- Salt and black pepper
- Optional: squeeze of lemon or a sprinkle of paprika

How to make it:

1. Scrub the potatoes clean but leave the skins on. Place in a pan of cold, lightly salted water and bring to a boil.
2. Reduce the heat and simmer for 15 to 20 minutes, or until the potatoes are fork-tender.
3. Drain well and let them steam dry for a minute.
4. Toss the warm potatoes with olive oil, chopped dill, and a pinch of salt and pepper. Add lemon or paprika if using.
5. Serve warm or at room temperature.

Neutral pairing tip:

You can serve this with steamed green beans or a handful of

rocket. Keep it green and light. No eggs, no fish, no dairy, let the potatoes stand on their own.

Fruit timing:
Avoid fruit with or directly after this meal. If you want fruit, have it on its own at least two hours later or 30 minutes before.

Storage:
Keeps well in the fridge for up to two days. Reheat gently or serve cold as part of a salad.

Why it works for the Hay Diet:
Potatoes are your carbohydrate. The herbs, oil, and optional veg are neutral. No protein means smoother digestion and less bloating.

Vegetable Soup with Pearl Barley

What you need:

- 60g pearl barley, rinsed
- 1 tablespoon olive oil
- 1 small onion, chopped
- 1 carrot, diced
- 1 celery stick, diced
- 1 courgette, chopped
- 2 garlic cloves, minced
- 750ml vegetable stock (low salt)
- 1 bay leaf
- Salt and black pepper

How to make it:

1. Heat the olive oil in a large pan. Add the onion, carrot, and celery. Cook over medium heat for 5 to 7 minutes until softened.

2. Add the garlic and courgette, and cook for another 2 minutes.

3. Stir in the barley, bay leaf, and stock. Bring to a boil, then reduce heat and simmer gently for 30 to 35 minutes, or until the barley is tender.

4. Season with salt and pepper to taste. Remove the bay leaf before serving.

Neutral pairing tip:
You don't need anything on the side. If you want to make it stretch further, serve with a cucumber and dill salad dressed in lemon juice, just don't add bread or cheese.

Fruit timing:
No fruit with or after this. Wait at least two hours before eating fruit, or enjoy it 30 minutes before your meal instead.

Storage:
This soup keeps well for up to three days in the fridge. It also freezes nicely. Reheat gently on the hob with a splash of water if needed.

Why it works for the Hay Diet:
The pearl barley is your starch. The vegetables, herbs, and stock are neutral. It's a proper one-bowl meal that's easy on digestion and doesn't leave you feeling stuffed or foggy afterwards.

Rice Noodles with Pak Choi and Ginger Broth

What you need:

- 60g dry rice noodles

- 500ml water or light vegetable stock

- 1 head of pak choi, halved or sliced

- 2 spring onions, chopped

- 1 thumb-sized piece of fresh ginger, peeled and finely sliced

- 1 garlic clove, minced

- 1 tablespoon tamari or light soy sauce

- 1 teaspoon sesame oil

- A dash of lemon juice or rice vinegar

How to make it:

1. In a saucepan, bring the water or stock to a gentle boil. Add the sliced ginger, garlic, and spring onions. Simmer for 5 minutes to infuse the broth.

2. Add the tamari and a squeeze of lemon juice or vinegar.

3. Drop in the pak choi and simmer for another 2–3 minutes until just wilted.

4. In a separate pan, cook the rice noodles according to the packet instructions, then drain and rinse under cold water to stop them sticking.

5. Divide the noodles into a bowl and ladle the broth and vegetables over the top. Drizzle with sesame oil and serve hot.

Neutral pairing tip:
Avoid adding tofu or egg to this broth if you're keeping it in the carb category. If you want to turn it into a protein meal, skip the noodles and add tofu instead.

Fruit timing:

Do not follow this meal with fruit. If you want fruit, have it 30 minutes before or two hours after.

Storage:

Store the broth and noodles separately. Broth will keep for two days in the fridge. Noodles are best used within 24 hours.

Why it works for the Hay Diet:

Rice noodles are the starch. Everything else, pak choi, ginger, garlic, tamari, is neutral. It's a warming, soothing meal that doesn't weigh you down or confuse your digestion.

Vegetable Stir-Fry with Brown Rice and Garlic-Sesame Dressing

What you need:

- 75g brown rice

- 1 tablespoon olive oil or sesame oil

- 1 small courgette, sliced into thin half-moons

- 1 carrot, julienned or grated

- 1 handful shredded cabbage

- 1 garlic clove, minced

- ½ teaspoon grated ginger

- 1 teaspoon rice vinegar

- A few sesame seeds for topping

- Salt and black pepper

How to make it:

1. Cook the brown rice in double the amount of water until tender, about 25 minutes. Drain and let it steam dry.

2. While the rice cooks, heat the oil in a pan or wok. Add the garlic and ginger, stir for 30 seconds, then add the carrot, courgette, and cabbage.

3. Stir-fry for 5 to 7 minutes until the veg are just tender but still bright. Add rice vinegar, salt, and pepper to taste.

4. Serve the rice topped with the stir-fried vegetables and a sprinkle of sesame seeds.

Neutral pairing tip:
If you want to bulk this out, add sliced cucumber or steamed bok choy on the side, both are neutral. Avoid any tofu or egg here; they'll turn this into a protein-carb mix.

Fruit timing:
Avoid fruit with or directly after this dish. Wait two hours before having fruit or eat it at least 30 minutes beforehand.

Storage:
This keeps well in the fridge for up to two days. Reheat the rice and veg gently on the hob or enjoy cold.

Why it works for the Hay Diet:
Brown rice provides the carbohydrate, and all vegetables and seasonings are neutral. There's no protein involved, so digestion stays smooth and focused.

Vegetable Fried Rice with Spring Onion and Sesame

This dish is a comforting classic, offering the savoury satisfaction of fried rice without any protein conflicts. It's quick to prepare and perfect for using up leftover rice.

What you need:

- 75g cooked brown rice (preferably chilled)

- 1 tablespoon sesame oil

- 1 small carrot, finely diced

- 1 celery stick, finely diced

- 2 spring onions, sliced

- 1 garlic clove, minced

- 1 teaspoon grated fresh ginger

- 1 tablespoon tamari or light soy sauce

- A pinch of white pepper

- Optional: a sprinkle of toasted sesame seeds

How to make it:

1. Heat the sesame oil in a wok or large frying pan over medium heat.

2. Add the garlic and ginger, sautéing for 30 seconds until fragrant.

3. Stir in the carrot and celery, cooking for 3–4 minutes until slightly softened.

4. Add the cooked rice, breaking up any clumps, and stir-fry for another 3–4 minutes until heated through.

5. Mix in the spring onions, tamari, and white pepper, stirring well to combine.

6. Serve hot, garnished with toasted sesame seeds if desired.

Neutral pairing tip:

Pair with a side of steamed greens like bok choy or a simple cucumber salad dressed with rice vinegar. Avoid adding tofu or eggs to keep it carbohydrate-focused.

Fruit timing:

Refrain from consuming fruit with or immediately after this meal. If desired, have fruit at least 30 minutes before or 2 hours after eating.

Storage:

Store leftovers in an airtight container in the refrigerator for up to 2 days. Reheat thoroughly before serving.

Why it works for the Hay Diet:

Brown rice serves as the carbohydrate base, while the vegetables and seasonings are neutral, ensuring proper food combining and optimal digestion.

Udon Noodle Soup with Miso and Greens

This light yet satisfying soup combines chewy udon noodles with a flavourful miso broth and fresh greens, making it an ideal meal for any time of day.

What you need:

- 80g dried udon noodles
- 500ml water
- 1 tablespoon white miso paste
- 1 teaspoon grated fresh ginger
- 1 garlic clove, minced
- 1 spring onion, sliced
- 1 handful of spinach or pak choi
- 1 teaspoon sesame oil
- Optional: a dash of tamari for extra flavour

How to make it:

1. Cook the udon noodles according to the package instructions. Drain and set aside.

2. In a saucepan, bring the water to a gentle simmer. Add the ginger, garlic, and miso paste, whisking until the miso dissolves.

3. Add the greens and simmer for 2–3 minutes until wilted.

4. Place the cooked noodles in a bowl and pour the hot broth over them.

5. Drizzle with sesame oil and garnish with sliced spring onion. Add tamari if desired.

Neutral pairing tip:

Enjoy this soup on its own or with a side of steamed vegetables. Avoid adding proteins like tofu or eggs to maintain proper food combining.

Fruit timing:

Do not consume fruit with or immediately after this meal. If desired, have fruit at least 30 minutes before or 2 hours after eating.

Storage:

Store the broth and noodles separately in the refrigerator for up to 2 days. Reheat the broth and combine with noodles just before serving.

Why it works for the Hay Diet:

Udon noodles provide the carbohydrate component, while the miso broth and vegetables are neutral, aligning with the Hay Diet's food combining guidelines.

Final Reminders for Using These Recipes

Before you start experimenting with these meals, keep a few core Hay Diet principles in mind. These aren't strict rules for the sake of being strict, they're what make the difference between a body that digests smoothly and one that stays stuck in discomfort.

- Always follow proper food combining: never mix protein and carbohydrates in the same meal.

- Use neutral vegetables to complete meals and bring in flavour, fibre, and balance.

- If you want fruit, have it on its own, between meals. Never eat fruit as a dessert.

- Most of these meals can be doubled or prepped in batches. The simpler your routine, the easier this becomes.

- Stay hydrated, but avoid drinking large amounts with meals. Let your stomach do its work undiluted.

Stick to these foundations, and these meals won't just help you feel full, they'll help you feel better. That's the whole point.

Chapter 11: tips for Long-Term Success

By now, you've seen how the Hay Diet works. You've learned the food combinations, started to feel the difference in your digestion, and maybe even noticed changes in your mood, your weight, your sleep. But here's where most people get stuck, not in the food itself, but in how they think about it.

If you still see this as a "diet," it'll always feel temporary. Something you're on until you're off again. Something to follow until a holiday comes up, or life gets busy, or motivation fades. And then you're back where you started.

That's not what this is meant to be.

This only starts to work in the long term when it stops feeling like a diet altogether. When it becomes just... how you eat. How you live.

You're not counting points. You're not weighing food. You're not cutting out entire food groups. You're just choosing to eat in a way that supports your body instead of fighting against it. And once you've experienced that calm after meals, once you've stopped waking up bloated or dragging through the day, it's hard to unlearn.

I always go back to this line:

"Once you understand the principles of the diet, and you start to lose weight and generally feel better, you will grow to love this way of eating."

That's exactly how it happened for me.

I didn't fall in love with it overnight. I didn't do everything right from the beginning. I had my moments of second-guessing, temptation, laziness. But the longer I stuck with it, the more obvious it became, my body worked better this way. I wasn't hungry all the time. I wasn't relying on caffeine to stay awake. I wasn't chasing food to fix how I felt. My meals did their job, and I could move on with my day.

That's the shift. When eating well no longer feels like a project. It's just part of your life now.

And once it becomes normal, you don't need willpower. You just keep doing what works

Daily Habits That Make It Stick

For this way of eating to last, it has to blend into your everyday life. That doesn't happen through motivation, it happens through rhythm. Through habits that work quietly in the background, without making everything harder.

The first thing I committed to was eating three proper meals a day. No in-between picking. No snacks out of boredom. Just breakfast, lunch, and dinner. Each one properly combined.

Once I found that rhythm, the guessing stopped. I wasn't grazing all day or reacting to hunger that didn't need to be there. I gave my body breaks between meals, and that space made everything smoother. My digestion felt steadier. My energy was more even. And food wasn't taking up so much headspace anymore.

The second habit was keeping fruit separate. I stopped throwing it in with breakfast or finishing a meal with it, and only had it between meals, never with them. Two hours after lunch, or an hour before the next meal. That one change stopped a lot of the gas and bloating I used to think was normal.

I also slowed down how I ate. Not just the chewing, but the pace of the whole meal. Before this, I was eating in the car, at my desk, while doing other things. That kind of rushed eating always left me feeling heavy or uncomfortable afterward. Now I sit down, even if it's just for ten minutes. I chew properly. I pay attention. Not because it's a rule, but because it feels better that way.

I keep a few things prepped, too. Boiled eggs in the fridge. A container of chopped vegetables. Cooked brown rice. Just the basics. That way, even when the day's packed or I get home late, I don't have to scramble. I already have something to work with.

And through all of this, I've kept one thing in mind: there's no need to chase perfection. If I mix something wrong or eat off-pattern, I don't spiral. I don't start over or get dramatic. I just go back to the routine with the next meal.

These habits aren't about discipline. They're about making this simple enough to keep going. When your meals have structure and your days aren't filled with food stress, this stops feeling like a "diet" altogether. It just becomes the way you eat.

It's one thing to follow the Hay Diet when you're at home, with a full fridge and a bit of time. But real life isn't always like that. You'll have days when you're rushed, travelling, eating out, or completely off your routine. And if you're not prepared for those moments, they're the ones that usually throw you off.

Over the years, I've found a few steady ways to keep the diet going when everything around me is unpredictable.

When I travel, I keep things neutral until I'm in control again. I stick to vegetables, olive oil, eggs, or simple salads, foods that don't cause issues on their own and give me breathing space until I can find proper meals that fit the structure.

On busy days, I make sure I've got something ready. That might be a boiled egg, a small tub of rice and veg, or even a plain fruit snack in between if the timing lines up. I don't rely on takeout or hope I'll figure it out later. I keep one or two fallback meals in mind that I know I can throw together without much effort.

And when I eat out, I follow the same rule I do at home: choose *either* protein or starch, not both. Then I look at the plate and decide what doesn't fit, and I leave it. I don't explain, I don't make it awkward. I've said I was full, or that something wasn't sitting well with me, or just pushed it to the side quietly.

That one line has saved me from countless poorly combined meals.

I am not saying you have to control each & every situation. But you need to learn how to stay steady when things get unpredictable. Because life *will* get in the way sometimes. That's not failure. It's just reality.

What matters is how you respond. Missing the mark once doesn't undo anything. You come back to your next meal. You stick to the pattern that works. That's what builds consistency, not doing it perfectly, but knowing how to return to it without making it dramatic.

This diet fits into your life if you let it. You don't need to fix every situation; you just need to make better choices more often than not. That's what makes it sustainable.

Staying Motivated

The hardest part isn't getting started. It's staying with it once the novelty wears off. After the first few weeks, once the changes become routine, the mind starts drifting. You forget how bad your digestion used to feel. You stop noticing how different things are because the discomfort is no longer part of your daily life. That's when people tend to loosen up, and when old habits slowly start creeping back in.

So it helps to stop and think about *why* you started in the first place.

Maybe it was the constant bloating. Or waking up tired. Maybe it was that uncomfortable, sluggish feeling after meals. Or the frustration of doing everything "right" and still not feeling well. Whatever it was, don't lose sight of it. Keep it close.

Most of the progress that matters don't show up on a scale. It shows up in how your body feels, in how your clothes fit, in how your mood levels out throughout the day. That's what I call non-scale victories.

You'll start noticing:

- Less bloating after meals

- Better sleep without needing to "crash"

- Regular digestion without discomfort

- Fewer cravings that come out of nowhere

- A clearer head, less fog, more energy that lasts

These are the signs that your system is working with you again, not against you.

Some people find it helpful to keep a small notebook or a phone note where they track what's changing. It doesn't have to be obsessive, just short reminders of what's improving. It's easy to forget progress once it becomes normal.

You don't need a big support group or to announce it to the world, but it does help to tell someone. A partner, a sibling, a friend, someone who knows what you're doing and won't offer you dessert five minutes after dinner. That small bit of awareness from people around you makes it easier to stay on track.

What's surprised me most over the years is how simple this gets once it becomes part of your life. You are not being disciplined anymore. You are not trying to motivate yourself. It's just your routine now. The meals make sense. The digestion feels better. You stop reaching for the things that used to leave you uncomfortable, not because you're avoiding them, but because you genuinely don't want to go back to that feeling.

That's where this way of eating starts to hold.

Community & Encouragement

You've made it this far because something inside you wanted to feel better. Not just for a week or for a goal weight, but for good. And if you've felt even a glimpse of what this diet can do for your digestion, your energy, or your clarity, then you already know, this isn't theory. It's real.

This isn't a trend. It's not some flash-in-the-pan wellness fad that'll be replaced by something flashier in six months. The Hay Diet has been around for decades, and it's worked quietly, consistently, for people like me who stuck with it. Not because it promised magic, but because it *delivered results* that actually lasted.

Remember, I'm living proof that this diet works. All you have to decide is, am I going to follow Robert down the same path he went down 35 years ago?

That's is not a self-praise. That's the whole point of this book.

You're not doing this alone. If you have questions, if you hit a wall, if you want to share what's changed for you, I want to hear it. I'm not a doctor. I'm not a health influencer. I'm someone who found a system that helped and stuck with it. And if you're reading this book, you've already taken the first steps on that same path.

Reach out. Ask what's unclear. Share what's worked for you. Whether it's a message, an email, or something you pass on to someone else who's struggling with the same gut problems, this works better when it's shared.

You can contact me directly at **_haydietnew@outlook.com_**. I'd love to hear how you're getting on, answer your questions, or just offer a bit of encouragement if you're finding the transition tricky.

This isn't just about food combining. It's about reclaiming how you feel after meals, how you move through the day, and how you take care of your body without relying on diets, pills, or confusion.

You've already started. Now it's about carrying it forward, one meal at a time, with a bit of awareness, and a lot less stress than you probably thought it would take.

Chapter 12: Final Thoughts

I know how strange this way of eating can feel when you first begin. It's not like the plans we're used to. You're not cutting out food groups, counting points, or weighing every bite. You're not being told what time to eat or how much. You're just combining food differently, and that can feel almost too simple at first.

But simple doesn't mean weak. It means clear. And once the body starts responding, you begin to realise this isn't just another diet. It's a reset. Not just for your stomach, but for how you think about meals, how you move through the day, and how you feel inside your own skin.

That first week or two might be a little awkward. You'll probably forget some rules, mix things without meaning to, feel unsure about what to eat when you're out. That's all part of the process. I went through it myself. I didn't get it right from day one. But I didn't stop, either.

You're not aiming for perfect. You're just learning a rhythm. And if you give it a bit of time, if you stick with it long enough to feel what it does for you, it stops being a set of rules and starts becoming your normal.

This diet works. I'm not telling you that because I read it somewhere. I'm telling you that because I've lived it. For 35 years.

I didn't stay on this diet for three decades because I was trying to be disciplined. I stayed on it because it worked. Quietly. Day after day. Once the bloating stopped, once my digestion started moving properly, once my meals left me feeling calm instead of uncomfortable, I had no reason to go back.

Will power alone will not cut it. You need to experiment and learn what suits your body, and then not unlearn it. Once you begin, you will start to notice which combinations leave you feeling heavy. Which ones sit cleanly. You don't need a chart after a while, you just feel it. And that becomes the guide.

I've been the same weight, 162 pounds, for 35 years. No calorie tracking. No exercise obsession. Just food that works with my body, not against it. I feel better in my sixties than I did in my forties. I wake up with no aches or pains. I don't drag through the day. My meals do what they're supposed to, fuel me, not fight me.

And I'm not saying that to impress you. I'm saying it because this isn't some theory. It's real. I've lived every part of what you've just read.

You don't need to do everything perfectly. You just need to stick with it long enough for the results to show up. That's where the mind-set shifts. When you're no longer trying to follow the diet, you're just eating the way that keeps you well.

If you've made it this far through the book, you've already taken the most important step, you've paid attention. Not to noise, not to trends, but to what's been quietly working in the background for years.

Now it's your turn to test it.

Don't wait for the perfect time. Just give it 10 days. That's what I did. I changed how I combined my meals, and I didn't look back. I lost two stone in three months. But it wasn't the weight that kept me going. It was how I felt. The clarity after meals. The ease in my body. The feeling that food wasn't a fight anymore.

I am not asking you to follow every detail to the book but what I would ask of you is to give your body a break from the mess. give it time to reset. Let it do what it was built to do, digest cleanly, use what it needs, and move the rest along.

You must make the decision: **AM I WORTH IT?**

That's what it comes down to in the end. Not motivation. Not goals. Just that one question.

And when you give your body the chance to answer, it usually does.

And I'll say this once again, if you've followed this all the way through and started making changes, big or small, I'd like to hear how it's going. You're not a stranger reading a manual. You're someone on the same road I've been walking for decades. And if something I've learned can help you, I'd rather you ask than struggle in silence.

If you've got a question, send it. If you want to share what has changed for you, even just one meal that felt better than usual, I'll read it. And if enough people want to stay in touch, maybe we'll build something simple. A way to keep the encouragement going.

You already know the principles. You know how to combine foods. You know what works and what gets in the way. Now it's up to you.

You can't change the past. But you *can* change what you put on your plate today. And sometimes, that's where everything else begins.

I wish you a smooth journey and a healthy & happy life.

With love,

-Robert

Printed in Dunstable, United Kingdom

70863359R00074